Dr Ante Bilić
liječnik - stomatolog

Ante Bilić
09.02.1981

Tooth Movement with Removable Appliances

J D Muir

BDS, UBirm, LDS, DOrth, FDS, RCSEng
Consultant Orthodontist
Staffordshire Area Health Authority

R T Reed

BDS, UGlasg, DOrth, RCSEng, FDS, RCPSGlasg
Consultant Orthodontist
Hampshire Area Health Authority

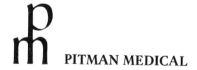

PITMAN MEDICAL

First published 1979

Catalogue Number 21 2449 81

Pitman Medical Publishing Co Ltd
P O Box 7, Tunbridge Wells,
Kent, TN1 1XH, England

Associated Companies

UNITED KINGDOM
Pitman Publishing Ltd, London
Focal Press Ltd, London

CANADA
Copp Clark Ltd, Toronto

USA
Fearon Pitman Publishers Inc, California
Focal Press Inc, New York

AUSTRALIA
Pitman Publishing Pty Ltd, Carlton

NEW ZEALAND
Pitman Publishing NZ Ltd, Wellington

British Library Cataloguing in Publication Data
Muir, J D
    Tooth movement with removable appliances.
    1. Orthodontic appliances
    I. Title   II. Reed, R T
    617.6'43'0028   RK527

    ISBN 0-272-79424-4

Set in 11 on 13 pt. IBM Journal by
Gatehouse Wood Ltd, Cowden, Kent
Printed by offset-lithography and bound
in Great Britain at The Pitman Press, Bath

Contents

Melius est reprehendant nos grammatici quam non intelligant populi.

St Augustine (354–430).

It is better that the professors should reproach us than that the people not understand.

Preface

Many orthodontic textbooks have been written by those who are primarily teachers rather than clinicians. As a result texts, which are in other ways excellent, fail to speak with authority on the practicalities of treatment.

We have set out to produce a book which will serve as a useful chairside guide to the practitioner rather than a comprehensive reference work, limiting ourselves to describing appliances which we have used and found to be effective.

A practical guide must necessarily omit certain subjects. Functional appliances, a study in their own right, have been excluded. Details of patient examination and treatment planning are largely outside the scope of this book, but because appliance design is intimately related to planned tooth movements, emphasis has been placed on space assessment, anchorage control and measurement of progress. We have omitted reference lists and bibliography. So many sources of practical information are not in print but derive from personal communications from our past teachers and our colleagues. We are glad to have this opportunity of thanking them publicly.

Regardless of the number of trained specialists and the popularity of fixed appliances it seems likely that much treatment will be carried out by the interested practitioner rather than the specialist. We believe that removable appliance techniques can make a valuable contribution to the provision of an orthodontic service. They may offer neither the precise tooth movements nor the adaptability of fixed appliances but, used in selected cases, they can provide good results. There is also a wider range of cases in which circumstances may prevent the complex treatment which would be necessary to achieve perfection, but where treatment with a removable appliance may provide a result which pleases the patient and is acceptable to the orthodontist. Such a result, though falling short of the ideal, can be regarded as a success if it is the fulfilment of a well considered treatment plan efficiently executed.

In order to use any appliance to the best advantage it is essential for the operator to select appropriate cases, to match appliance design to the required tooth movement and to maintain effective control of the clinical treatment. We hope that this book will assist the practitioner in achieving these ends.

J.D.M.
R.T.R.

CHAPTER 1

The Scope
of Removable Appliances

A removable appliance is one which, by definition, can be easily removed from the mouth. This must not be thought to imply that such appliances are intended for part-time wear. With the exception of certain functional appliances and retainers, removable appliances will only perform their tasks satisfactorily if they are worn continuously. This means that not only must the patient be enthusiastic and co-operative but that the operator has a duty so to design and construct the appliances that they can be readily tolerated by such a patient.

For this reason it is important that the appliance is not only easy to remove but also easy to insert, that it should stay firmly in the correct position in the mouth and that it should be comfortable to wear. It should be designed to avoid causing pain or unnecessary discomfort and should not be so bulky or complex that it interferes seriously with speech and eating. Only in these circumstances can we reasonably insist upon full-time wear.

The vast majority of removable appliances are used in the upper arch but a small number of useful movements can also be carried out in the lower arch. A keen patient may be prepared to wear an upper and lower appliance at the same time but this constitutes a great bulk in the mouth and is usually not advisable. The main indication for a removable appliance is to provide treatment in the upper arch when the lower is to have:

1. no treatment
2. treatment by extractions only
3. treatment with a fixed appliance.

This is an appropriate moment to stress that removable

1

and fixed appliances are not mutually exclusive. The Hawley type of retainer is used by many orthodontists who would class themselves as using only fixed appliances, and it is not uncommon for certain movements to be carried out with a removable appliance during the course of fixed appliance treatment, e.g. the initial retraction of mesially inclined canines.

Similarly the scope of removable appliances may be extended considerably by the use of one or two bands for the attachment of whips, hooks, or extra oral traction.

Despite this it must be stressed that removable appliances do not constitute a 'complete treatment philosophy'. Some tooth movements may be carried out with ease, some with difficulty and others not at all. Obviously the orthodontist can only hope for success if he selects cases which are suitable for treatment with removable appliances, i.e. cases requiring the type of tooth movements which these appliances can carry out.

TOOTH MOVEMENT

The histology of tooth movement is beyond the scope of this book but a useful analogy to the behaviour of a tooth may be obtained by comparing it with a post embedded in thick mud. This is obviously not an accurate comparison but it will serve our purpose. If pressure is applied to the post it can be readily tilted in any direction. An ill-defined fulcrum is set up and the embedded end of the post will move in the opposite direction to that in which the pressure is applied. If the post is grasped firmly with both hands the range of possible movements is much greater. It can be rotated, moved bodily, or the embedded base can be moved more than the top. It can also be pushed further into the mud or pulled out.

Simple Tilting Movements

A removable appliance most commonly delivers its force through a single point of contact where a spring touches the tooth. Simple tilting movements can be easily carried out and teeth may be tipped mesially, distally, buccally or lingually. As in the analogy of the post the apex will move in the opposite direction. It has traditionally been held that the fulcrum of rotation is about one third of the root length

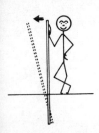

Tilting movements are readily carried out with light pressures.

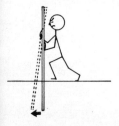

Complex movements are difficult to carry out. More control is required.

from the apex but it seems probable that it is often much nearer the crown than this. It can be seen that retraction of an inclined tooth which requires uprighting (e.g. a mesially inclined canine which must be retracted) can give a good result. If a tooth which is already at the correct inclination must be moved then some degree of tilting will have to be accepted. If a tooth is already inclined and has to be moved further in the direction of its inclination (e.g. a retroclined canine which has to be further retracted) then a removable appliance is usually unsuitable.

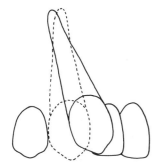

A mesially inclined canine will tilt readily into a good position.

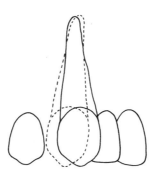

The tilting which results from slight distal movement of an upright canine may be acceptable.

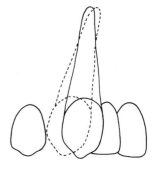

A canine which is already distally inclined would tilt more severely during retraction.

Other Movements

Movements which in the analogy of the stick required the grip of both hands pose greater difficulties. A force couple is required. In theory force can be applied by two wires or by a wire in conjunction with the base plate. Unfortunately the degree of flexibility of the wires necessary to permit insertion and removal of the appliance, and to deliver a light force, usually makes it impossible to keep the force applied constantly in the correct position.

Rotation

It is frequently held that removable appliances cannot correct rotations. This is not strictly true. Central incisors or large lateral incisors can often be corrected if the problem is only a simple rotation of up to about 45°. Multiple rotations, more severe individual rotations, and those in teeth with crowns which are round in cross-section, e.g. premolars and canines, are impossible to correct with a removable appliance alone.

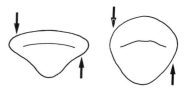

A force couple can be achieved on a flat tooth such as a central incisor. This is impossible on a canine or premolar.

3

The addition of a band to a single rotated tooth with a whip engaging on to part of the appliance (Chapter 11) will allow the correction of more severe rotations and also of canines and premolars. It is important, however, to check that the problem is simply a rotation. Many rotations have an associated apical malposition which may make the problem impossible without the control offered by full banded appliances. If an attempt is made to treat such a problem with a simple whip and band the tooth will tend to upright over its apex and will probably finish in the wrong position and at the wrong height.

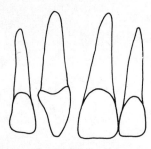

A severe rotation with the apex in a normal position.

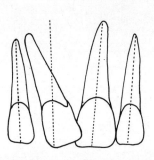

In this example the rotation is less severe but is combined with apical displacement.

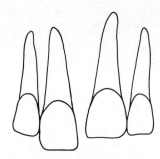

Treatment by simple means is unsatisfactory.

Intrusive Movements

Deliberate intrusive movement of a single tooth is hardly ever required. It would be technically possible to deliver the force although it would tend to unseat the appliance.

Extrusive Movements

These provide another example of the sort of movement which is impossible by means of a simple removable appliance alone but which can be facilitated by the attachment of a hook, either on a band or directly bonded to the enamel. It may be particularly useful when a tooth has been surgically uncovered following failure to erupt.

Apical and Bodily Movements

Generally speaking these are not possible with removable appliances. Designs have been demonstrated recently which successfully produce such movements but they are limited to the upper labial segment and depend upon having the teeth already aligned and on the use of enthusiastic head-gear. They may be useful in selected cases but are beyond the scope of this book.

Arch Levelling

This is usually not possible with a removable appliance. The chief exception is the use of an anterior bite plane in a growing patient to permit molar extrusion and so flatten out an exaggerated curve of Spee in the lower arch (Chapter 2).

Space Closure

The presence of a rigid base plate makes removable appliances inefficient at generalized space closure and their use for this purpose must usually be limited to carrying out local movements and to cases where overjet reduction is required as a contribution to space closure.

ANCHORAGE

The control of anchorage is an important consideration in tooth movement by any system and removable appliances are no exception.

Anchorage is a concept easy to understand but hard to define and the definitions found in many textbooks are unsatisfactory. Beginners sometimes confuse anchorage with retention (i.e. the mechanism by which an appliance is held in the mouth). Fortunately most orthodontists have at least some idea of what they mean by the word and it is certainly important that anyone carrying out tooth movement should understand the concept and control of anchorage.

Newton's third law of motion states that every force has an equal and opposite reaction. This is of obvious relevance in orthodontics because teeth are moved by the application of force. The reaction to this force will usually fall upon other teeth which are themselves capable of movement.

We consider anchorage to mean the resistance to movement offered by the teeth used to deliver an orthodontic force. Removable appliances rely upon intra-maxillary traction, i.e. anchorage is obtained from within the same arch. In some circumstances anchorage may be reciprocal. This means that the anchorage requirements of two teeth

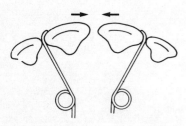

The equal and opposite movements provide an example of true reciprocal anchorage.

or groups of teeth cancel each other out. Examples of this are provided by the approximation of two central incisors or during the closure of excess space by the reduction of an overjet and the forward movement of upper buccal segments.

More usually we wish to move certain teeth whilst leaving the rest of the arch unchanged.

The force necessary to carry out a simple tipping movement on a single rooted tooth is usually said to be in the region of 30 to 50 g. There is a threshold of perhaps about 20 g below which movement does not occur.

Our problem is to deliver sufficient force to move the required teeth while ensuring that the reactionary force, when divided among the anchor teeth, is insufficient to cause movement.

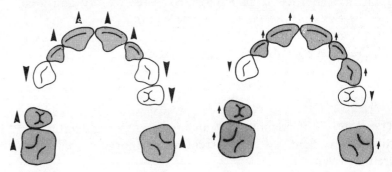

The reaction to heavy forces applied simultaneously to too many teeth is likely to produce forward movement of the anchor teeth.

A light force applied to one tooth in each quadrant throws less strain on the anchor teeth and will minimize their forward movement.

Except where very minor tooth movement is being carried out some movement of the anchorage teeth frequently occurs. This is described as anchorage loss. Forward movement of buccal teeth occurs very readily particularly in the upper arch. This is frequently seen when physiological mesial drift occurs after premolar extractions have been carried out, even when appliances have not been used. In cases where space is not critical some anchorage loss may be acceptable. In other cases it may be vital that anchorage loss does not occur.

Anchorage may be conserved in two main ways:

1. Keeping Forces Light

Removable appliances conserve anchorage well because they allow simple tipping movements of the teeth which require the lightest pressures. The reactionary force can be reduced by limiting the number of teeth moved. Only one buccal tooth per quadrant should be moved in the same direction at any one time and when an overjet is to be reduced the incisors should not be moved palatally while other teeth are being retracted. Nevertheless it is unwise to assume that anchorage loss will be completely avoided merely by the use of light forces.

2. Increasing the Resistance of the Anchor Teeth

The Base Plate

The resistance offered by the fit of the base plate against the teeth and mucosa contributes to the good anchorage offered by removable appliances. This may be maximized by keeping the acrylic fitted around as many teeth as possible.

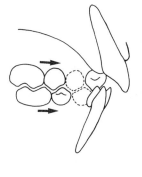

Cuspal Interlock

It seems likely that good cuspal interlock with the teeth of the opposing arch will offer added resistance to any anchorage loss. A problem, however, is that extractions in the opposing arch may allow the interlocked teeth to move mesially together. Further, when bite planes of any sort are used, cuspal interlock ceases to be effective.

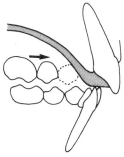

The helpful effects of cuspal interlock may be eliminated by lower extractions or the use of bite planes.

The Inclined Bite Plane

It is often claimed that the addition of an inclined anterior bite plane to an upper removable appliance will reinforce the anchorage by transmitting a distal thrust from the lower incisors when the patient occludes. It seems more likely that it will merely encourage the patient to posture the mandible forwards and in some cases it might cause proclination of the lower incisors. We think that it is wiser to reduce over-bites by the use of a flat anterior bite plane and to use more reliable methods of anchorage reinforcement in cases where this is necessary.

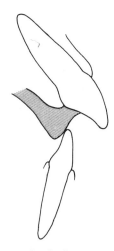

The Labial Bow

It is held in several textbooks that a labial bow placed incisally on the anterior teeth will prevent their proclination as a result of forward force applied through the acrylic base plate during the retraction of canines. In theory this might seem sensible. The acrylic and the labial wire should set up a

The use of an inclined bite plane makes no worthwhile contribution to anchorage.

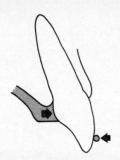

The traditional textbook view claims that the significant vertical separation between the palatal acrylic and the labial wire increases the anchorage value of the incisor teeth by establishing a rotational force couple.

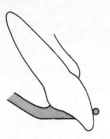

The saggital section of a model demonstrates the minimal vertical separation of wire and acrylic.

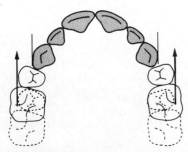

Forward movement of the buccal teeth produces prominence of the second premolars unless the arch width is reduced.

force couple which resists the forward tilting of the incisors and permits only their bodily forward movement. The anchorage value of these teeth to the appliance should thus be greatly increased.

In practice there is often very little vertical separation between the acrylic and the labial wire. In addition a long labial bow is too flexible to remain securely in the correct position. A short fitting wire around two or more upper incisors would be more rigid but it seems probable that its main contribution to anchorage would be made by improving retention and holding the appliance in tight contact with the teeth and mucosa.

Intermaxillary Traction

Again this has little practical application in removable appliance treatment. Traction might occasionally be used from a removable appliance, perhaps to support a lower fixed sectional arch, but this would be more for the benefit of the fixed appliance than the removable one.

Extra Oral Traction

This is the surest and most useful method of improving anchorage in a removable appliance. It can be applied in a wide variety of ways which will be dealt with in a later chapter. It is well tolerated and can extend considerably the scope of removable appliance treatment.

Deliberate Loss of Anchorage

Unless good anchorage reinforcement is being employed any major tooth movement will usually involve some slight shift of the anchor teeth. In certain treatments, however, extractions may be necessary but may consequently produce excessive space. In these cases forward movement of the buccal segments is desirable. Removable appliances do not carry this out particularly well because the base plate limits the necessary re-adaptation of the arch shape as space is closed. If anchorage is to be lost intentionally then provision must be made for narrowing the width of the arch to facilitate forward movement of the cheek teeth.

CONCLUSIONS

A removable appliance is less flexible than a fixed appliance; not only physically, in that it has a rigid base plate, but also in its adaptability. It is frequently possible to change the effect of a full banded appliance completely, e.g. by modifying an arch wire or altering elastic traction. By contrast a removable appliance is designed to carry out a small number of pre-determined tasks. Minor alterations may require considerable laboratory or chairside time; major ones may require total reconstruction of the appliance. It is important, therefore, that cases are selected carefully for removable appliance treatment. As with any other orthodontic treatment it is necessary to have a patient who is receiving regular dental care and has a good standard of oral hygiene and a healthy mouth. It is also necessary that a patient is keen to have treatment and is prepared to co-operate in the correct wearing and cleaning of the appliance.

Case Selection for Removable Appliance Therapy

Indications

1. The skeletal pattern should not be far removed from Class I. The increased or reversed overjet should be due mainly to changes in incisor inclination.
2. It should be possible to treat each arch individually. For example, the upper arch might be treated with removable appliances and the lower either with extractions only, no treatment or a simple fixed appliance.
3. Any individually malpositioned teeth should have their apices fairly well in line.
4. Planned extractions should allow tipping movements to correct the malocclusion.
5. Faults of bucco-lingual occlusion should be associated with a mandibular displacement. For example a unilateral crossbite of the posterior teeth.
6. Extractions should provide slight excess space or just sufficient space. Removable appliances are inefficient at space closure.

Contra-indications

1. A noticeable skeletal discrepancy exists.
2. There is a need to correlate treatment in both upper and lower arches. For example anchorage problems requiring

9

intermaxillary traction and more severe discrepancies in arch width or shape.

3. The presence of apical malpositions, severe or multiple rotations.

4. Bodily movements are required.

5. The presence of vertical discrepancies such as a deep overbite, an open bite or height discrepancies between teeth.

6. Space problems exist, for example severe crowding or excess of space.

In general the points made in this book refer to upper appliances although many are also relevant to lower appliances. Lower removable appliances are dealt with specifically in Chapter 7.

In the following chapters we shall deal with the design and construction of the component parts of removable appliances.

CHAPTER 2

Principles of Design:
The Acrylic Component

The body of a removable appliance consists mainly of the base plate which is made of acrylic resin. It can, if necessary, be extended and built up to form bite planes which will have an active influence on tooth position.

THE BASE PLATE

The base plate has two functions. Firstly it acts as a foundation into which the retaining clasps and active components of the appliance, such as springs and screws, are embedded. Secondly it contributes to the anchorage during the course of active tooth movement. It must provide a sufficient thickness of acrylic for the attachment of springs and retentive wirework but otherwise should be kept as thin as will be compatible with strength. The recommended thickness of the base plate is generally quoted as that of one sheet of modelling wax. In practice thicker base plates are often used satisfactorily but it is important that the acrylic should not be grossly thickened or the appliance may be difficult to wear, particularly during the initial adaptation period. The base plate should cover most of the hard palate and, while it may be trimmed away to permit movement or eruption of individual teeth, it should fit closely around the necks of those teeth which are not to be moved. The acrylic usually finishes across the vault of the palate just distal to the first molars.

Construction

The base plate is constructed on the model after completion of the wirework and boxing in of palatal springs. Conventionally heat-cured acrylic resins have been used. The springs are boxed in with plaster and a wax plate is built up and then flasked and processed in the same manner as for a denture. In recent years there has been a great increase in the use of 'cold cure' acrylic with a resultant economy of laboratory time. When this technique is used palatal springs are waxed rather than plastered in and other springs and clasps are secured in place with a dab of wax applied on the buccal side of the teeth. After the application of a separating medium the base plate is built up by the addition alternately of polymer powder and monomer liquid using a small plastic 'puffer' bottle and a glass dropper, respectively. If the model is tilted during this process the base plate can be built up in sections without unduly increasing the thickness of the appliance in the palatal vault. The model is placed in warm water in a pressure flask for a few minutes and this produces a non-porous acrylic which may be trimmed and finished in the normal manner. Several commercial brands of acrylic are now produced specifically for orthodontic purposes and almost all removable appliances used by the authors are constructed by a 'cold cure' technique. These appliances have proved entirely satisfactory in use. It is probably an advantage to use a transparent acrylic resin as areas of pressure can then be detected with the appliance in the mouth. Apart from the saving in time a particular advantage of this method is that the model can be retrieved intact in most cases. This often proves useful if the appliance has subsequently to be repaired or modified. Any possible distortion of the wirework during flasking and de-flasking is also eliminated.

Anchorage

The base plate makes an important contribution to the preservation of anchorage. It achieves this in two ways. First, teeth in addition to those which carry clasps can contribute to the anchorage through the close fit of the acrylic around their necks. The acrylic should fit around as many teeth as possible. An exception to this rule is that when first molars are being clasped it is usually better not to extend the acrylic around the second molars. The appliance is better tolerated when it does not extend this far distally and the second molars are frequently incompletely erupted and able to contribute little to anchorage.

The second way in which the base plate can contribute to

anchorage is through the contact of the appliance with the mucosa of the vault of the palate, particularly that part which has a significant vertical inclination. In this respect removable appliances have a distinct advantage over fixed appliances because they can bring the basal bone into the anchorage in addition to teeth which may be banded or clasped. The effect will only occur if the appliance is constructed so that it will be held in firm contact with the palate during wear. A removable appliance which is supported only by Adams' clasps on first molar teeth is unlikely to be effective in this way as it can readily slide downwards and forwards while the anchor teeth move mesially during anchorage loss. Adequate retention of the appliance anteriorly is essential if the base plate is to be firmly applied to the mucosa so that it can transmit any forward component of force from the appliance to the basal bone underlying it.

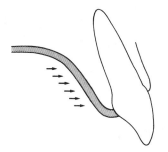

The palatal mucosa can offer considerable resistance to forward movement of the base plate.

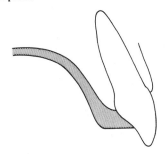

The base plate extended to form a bite plane.

ACTIVE COMPONENTS OF THE ACRYLIC

The base plate may be thickened or extended locally to form bite planes which will have an active effect on tooth position.

The Anterior Bite Plane

A common modification of the basic acrylic palate is the addition of an anterior bite plane. This takes the form of a thickened platform of acrylic, palatal to the upper incisors, on which the lower incisors can occlude leaving the posterior teeth out of occlusion.

Clinical Application

An anterior bite plane can be used to provide temporary relief of cuspal lock for the correction of bucco-lingual abnormalities in the buccal segments, but the chief use of an anterior bite plane is to bring about correction of an increased incisal overbite in a typical Class II malocclusion. If the operator is skilled and the patient is co-operative such a bite plane can be clinically very effective, but it is important to understand the way in which its effect is achieved.

It has been shown that overbite reduction produced by a removable appliance is only relative and is due largely to over-eruption of the buccal teeth which have been taken out of occlusion. There is little lower incisor intrusion. Because the overbite is reduced by molar extrusion the mandible must rotate downwards and backwards tending to increase the

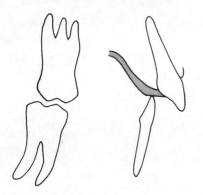

Mandibular rotation increases the face height and moves B point backwards.

facial height and produce a posterior movement of *B* point relative to *A* point. For minimal Class II cases which are suited to removable appliance treatment this is probably of limited clinical significance, but anterior bite planes should be used with circumspection in the treatment of more severe Class II cases with marked skeletal discrepancies or where there is an increased lower facial height. In such cases more sophisticated appliance techniques are advisable.

Construction and Adjustment of Anterior Bite Planes

It is difficult to provide the technician with accurate information to construct a suitable bite plane which can be fitted without chairside adjustment. Commonly the laboratory supplies an appliance with a bite plane which is too thick and which extends too far back. After fitting and preliminary inspection the appliance can be adapted as follows:

Correction of the height. Articulating paper should be used to aid the reduction of the bite plane until the posterior teeth are separated by from 1 to 2 mm. A separation of this degree will permit the necessary overbite reduction. At the same time it is possible for the patient to masticate food in a reasonably efficient manner and so to wear the appliance on a full-time basis. Undoubtedly one of the commonest errors in removable appliance treatment is the use of an anterior bite plane of too great a vertical dimension which separates the teeth to such a degree that it is difficult for the patient to eat with the appliance in place. This usually means that overbite reduction is very slow or totally unsuccessful.

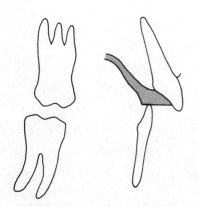

The anterior bite plane should separate the molars by no more that 1 to 2 mm.

Horizontal adjustment. The surface of the bite plane should be approximately parallel to the occlusal plane. It should also be horizontal when viewed from the front. Ideally the occlusal load should be spread over all six lower anterior teeth but the varying levels of the incisal edges and cusps may dictate a compromise. The aim must be to achieve a reasonable occlusal table on which the lower anterior teeth can function and yet to improve any irregularity in the height of these teeth as treatment proceeds. When the vertical adjustment has been carried out articulating paper can be used to make the final registration with the teeth closing in centric relation. Acrylic distal to the marks representing the incisal edges of the lower teeth should be removed. The

A bite plane of excessive thickness makes the appliance more difficult to wear.

14

redundant acrylic will only interfere with tongue function and make it more difficult for the patient to speak with the appliance in place. Over extension distally is a common error which leads to rejection of the appliance.

Finally the trimmed bite plane may be polished. When the appliance is finished in a nearby laboratory it is probably best left with a matt finish such as may be produced by pumice powder. If the finishing is carried out in the surgery then stones will probably give a sufficiently smooth finish to be comfortable.

Adjustments of the bite plane during treatment. If the appliance is fitted in the manner described and then worn full-time overbite reduction should be visible by the first visit a month later. This is especially true of growing patients.

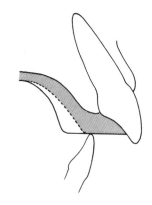

Unnecessary posterior extension of the bite plane serves no useful purpose and encroaches on tongue space.

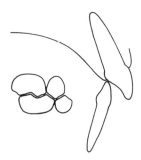

Incisor overbite is increased and complete.

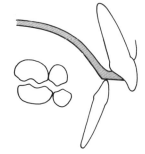

The bite plane produces molar separation when the appliance is fitted.

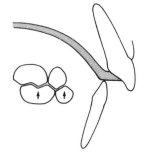

Continued wear allows the posterior teeth to erupt into occlusion.

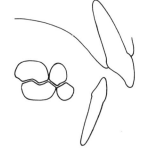

With the appliance removed the incisor overbite is now incomplete.

The molars should have over-erupted and by now be in full occlusion again with the appliance *in situ.* Facets representing functional contacts with the lower incisor teeth should be visible on the bite plane. Older patients may respond less rapidly to bite plane therapy. Difficulties are also sometimes encountered with other patients, particularly those who have a Class II, division 2 type of malocclusion with a very much increased overbite. If bite opening is progressing then the bite plane should be increased at this and subsequent visits as required. It is a relatively brief chairside procedure to add acrylic if the bite plane has been correctly adapted at the first appointment. A small quantity of cold cure acrylic is mixed in a Dappens pot and flowed on to the bite plane to a depth of about 1 mm, thereby eliminating the facets produced by the lower incisors. As soon as the acrylic is thickening it

15

may be placed for a few moments in a bowl of hot water to harden it to a point where it will only just indent with occlusal forces. The appliance is then returned to the mouth and the patient instructed to close gently in order to create slight indentations where the lower incisors occlude. This will allow the operator to check that the molars are again separated by 1 to 2 mm. No more trimming will be necessary and the patient may be dismissed until the next appointment. A cold cure acrylic with thixotropic properties is helpful as it has less tendency to spread from the bite plane in the newly mixed state. Such acrylics are produced chiefly for use in prosthetic dentistry.

By increasing the bite plane at each visit the overbite may be reduced and the curve of Spee levelled out. It is wise to open the bite a little further than would seem necessary to achieve a normal incisor overbite at the end of treatment. There is no danger of producing too much bite opening as any excess space will close rapidly if the bite plane is removed during the final stage of treatment.

Once sufficient overbite reduction has been achieved no further adjustments are necessary but the bite plane must be maintained on this and any subsequent appliances. Occasionally it may be necessary to continue overbite reduction with the second appliance especially when other tooth movements during the first stage of treatment are minimal.

It is important to maintain contact between the lower anterior teeth and upper bite plane even when the acrylic is trimmed during overjet reduction. For this reason trimming of the acrylic to allow incisor alignment and overjet reduction must be carried out with care. When a labial spring is to be activated to reduce the overjet it will be necessary to remove acrylic from behind the incisors to permit tooth movement. The palatal surfaces of these teeth should have 3 mm of acrylic removed from contact with them. It is sensible to draw a line with a grease pencil in this position with the appliance *in situ* and to check that this will not remove support from any of the lower anterior teeth. The appliance is then removed from the mouth and the acrylic trimmed back to this line.

The bite plane must then be undermined by trimming well up the palatal surface of the appliance tapering off at a minimum of about 7 mm beyond the gingival margin. If this is carried out correctly then it should be possible to see the

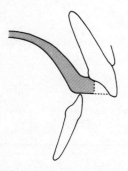

Trimming the acrylic Stage 1. An adequate platform remains for the lower incisors.

mucosa of the palate behind the upper incisors by direct inspection when the appliance is in place. At the same time sufficient of the horizontal surface of the bite plane will have been maintained to provide an occlusal table for the lower anterior teeth.

Errors in trimming removable appliances which carry anterior bite planes are common. Excessive trimming can permit the overbite to relapse before the overjet is successfully reduced. Inadequate palatal extension of the trimming may interfere with tooth movement by leaving acrylic in contact with the incisors at the gingival margin or with the related gingival tissue.

Only when the upper incisors are almost fully retracted should contact finally be lost between the acrylic and the lower anterior teeth by complete removal of the bite plane.

Posterior Bite Planes

It is occasionally necessary to cover the occlusal surfaces of the posterior teeth bilaterally to 'prop the bite' and so relieve cuspal lock while an anterior crossbite or a bucco-lingual abnormality is being corrected.

Clinical Application of Posterior Bite Planes

Incisor crossbite. Simple crossbites of incisor teeth can usually be treated without opening the bite despite the presence of a positive overbite. If a force is applied to the palatal surface of an instanding upper incisor it is usually possible for the mandible to displace forwards as this tooth moves. When sufficient tooth movement has occurred the mandible may return to centric relation, with normal incisor occlusion.

Bucco-lingual corrections. There are cases where crossbite correction cannot be assisted by a mandibular displacement. An example is provided by the attempted correction of an upper canine in crossbite. In such a case a suitable occlusal cover is most helpful. A further situation where a posterior bite plane is helpful is in the correction of a unilateral posterior crossbite associated with lateral mandibular displacement. As a general principle posterior bite planes should be avoided as they are probably the least acceptable of all aspects of removable appliance therapy. When they are

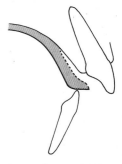

Trimming the arcylic Stage 2. The bite plane must be undermined well up the palatal surface.

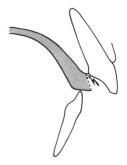

Incorrect trimming. Even though the acrylic is not touching the tooth, a small amount of movement will quickly re-establish contact. There is no space to accommodate the mucosa which is likely to become inflamed.

17

necessary they should be of minimum height commensurate with clinical need and should be used for the shortest possible time. It is wise to remove or reduce these bite planes as soon as possible.

Construction and Adjustment of Posterior Bite Planes

It is most important, when instructing the technician, to emphasize that the parts of clasps which cross the embrasure must not be incorporated into the acrylic covering the occlusal surfaces of the teeth. If this does occur then the flexibility and ease of adjustment of the retentive wirework will be severely limited. It is helpful to give the technician some indication of the height to which bite planes should be constructed. As in the case of anterior bite planes it is not easy to convey this information accurately and unless upper and lower working models are available for mounting on an articulator the appliance will probably require considerable modification at the chairside before it can be fitted.

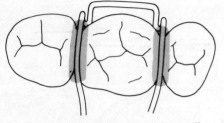

Clasp arms should be free from the acrylic of the bite plane where they cross the embrasure. This is achieved by adding wax before the acrylic is laid down.

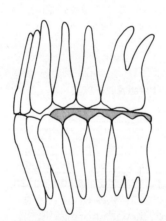

A common error, the bite planes are too thick and of uniform thickness, this props the bite posteriorly.

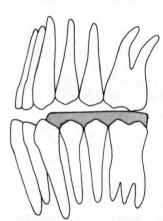

Correctly adjusted posterior bite plane giving even occlusal contact and minimal separation.

After the usual visual inspection and trial fit articulating paper can be used to aid reduction in the height of both bite planes. This reduction should be continued until the bite planes only just eliminate occlusal interference. This can mean that in some cases the bite planes will have been very much reduced over the posterior teeth. This is entirely acceptable since the need for minimum height to facilitate patient acceptance overrides the desire for strength and

18

resistance to occlusal wear. During the succeeding weeks such thin acrylic may frequently fracture or wear away but the duration of this phase of treatment should be short and the occlusal acrylic should survive for sufficient time to achieve the treatment objectives. Minor repairs can be carried out during treatment by the addition of cold cure acrylic as required. As soon as the bucco-lingual correction has been carried out the occlusal capping should be removed.

The above points relating to the adjustment of posterior bite planes apply equally when such bite planes are added to a lower appliance.

CHAPTER 3

Principles of Design:
Retentive and Passive Wirework

RETENTION

The term 'retention' is commonly used to describe the
mechanism whereby an appliance stays in the mouth. It is
unfortunate that the same term is in general use in orthodontics to denote the use of an appliance to maintain a
corrected tooth position. Fortunately the context in which
the word is used will usually avoid any ambiguity.

Good retention is important for a number of reasons.
Firstly it maintains the mechanical efficiency of the appliance
by ensuring that the springs are continuously held accurately
in position. Secondly because the appliance is a firm fit the
patient adapts to it more readily. Habit movements are
discouraged and the common initial difficulties with speech
and eating are minimized. Thirdly extra oral traction may be
added without risk of displacement. Finally the anchorage
contribution from the fit of the appliance against the teeth
and mucosa is maximized by preventing forward sliding of
the acrylic down the curvature of the palate.

The Adams' Clasp

Many clasps have been designed for use with removable
appliances but the advent of the universal or modified
arrowhead clasp, described by Adams, has rendered most
others obsolete. The description of this clasp and its construction given by Adams in his book* cannot be bettered,
but a number of points should be stressed:

*Adams, C.P. (1970) *Design and
Construction of Removable Orthodontic
Appliances.* Bristol: John Wright.

The Adams' Clasp Used on Molars

The clasp is constructed in 0.7 mm wire and can be adapted
for use on almost any tooth but is most commonly used on

first molars. A molar which has less than 4 mm of crown erupted generally gives poor retention. Even when the tooth is further erupted the clinical crown frequently fails to reveal parts of the anatomical crown which offer the best undercuts. In order to gain access to this undercut it is necessary to trim that part of the model representing the gingivae which obscures these areas. If this is correctly done the arrowhead will push the gingival margin aside as the appliance is inserted and engage the undercut. Inadequate trimming of the models, or the removal of plaster from the tooth rather than the gingivae, is a common reason for poorly fitting clasps. The clasp should not be active to any degree when in position. An undercut of 0.25 mm gives an adequate and optimal clasp. Clasps using deeper undercuts are more prone to distortion.

In adults sufficient undercut can usually be obtained without trimming the model and there may also be a very slight undercut on the palatal surfaces of the teeth which can provide useful added retention for the acrylic palate. During construction of the clasp the wire should be bent minimally and accurately. The clasp should fit the model closely where the embrasures are crossed to avoid damage by the opposing teeth. It should be noted that the position of the undercut is often not simply on the buccal aspect of the teeth but rather on the mesiobuccal and distobuccal corners and it is here that the arrowheads should engage. In addition to providing excellent retention the universal clasp offers other advantages:

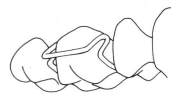

The clasp wire is adapted closely over the contact point and avoids damage from opposing teeth.

1. Its bridge provides a site to which the patient can apply pressure with the fingertips during removal of the appliance.

2. Auxilliary springs can be soldered to the bridge of the clasp.

3. Hooks can also be soldered to the clasp or bent in during construction to accept intermaxillary traction. It is nevertheless the opinion of the authors that for most cases requiring such traction fixed appliances are indicated.

4. Tubes can be soldered to the bridge of the clasp to accommodate a face bow for extra oral traction. It must be remembered, however, that such soldering, unless carefully carried out can lead to softening of the wire and thereby reduce the efficiency of the clasp.

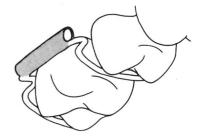

The soldered tube is attached gingivally to the bridge to avoid irritation of the buccal mucosa.

21

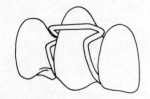

An Adams' clasp adapted for use on a canine.

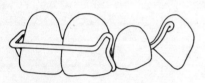

A double Adams' clasp on central incisors.

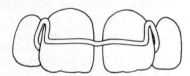

A less prominent version of the double incisor clasp.

* Dickson, G.C. and Wheatley, A.E. (1978) *An Atlas of Removable Orthodontic Appliances* Second Edition. Tunbridge Wells: Pitman Medical.

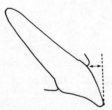

A clasping problem, proclined incisors provide too much undercut at the gingival margin.

The Adams' Clasp Used on Other Teeth

We have pointed out that the universal clasp is not only suited for use on molars. It is frequently useful to be able to clasp a premolar and so provide additional retention. Sometimes, where a molar is not available, a double clasp can be used across two adjacent premolars. A clasp on a canine is useful from time to time. Occasionally in the mixed dentition stage it may be necessary to clasp a deciduous first molar or canine and in such circumstances it is better to use 0.6 mm rather than 0.7 mm wire.

The clasp can also be used on incisors, either on an individual incisor or more commonly as a double clasp on upper central incisors. It is most suited to situations where the central incisors are upright or only mildly proclined. When there is no anterior spacing the arm of the clasp will pass over the top of the embrasure between the central and lateral incisors. The clasp is prone to breakage where it crosses this embrasure and the arm from the embrasure to the arrowhead is sometimes over long.

The clasp may be modified slightly by curving the bridge and flattening the arrowhead so that it stands out rather less from the teeth. Dickson and Wheatley describe such a modification in their laboratory manual.*

Limitations of the Adams' Clasp

On proclined incisors the universal clasp is not satisfactory. There is too much undercut labially and if the arrowheads engage only the correct amount of undercut then the bridge will be left perched on the most prominent part of the teeth near to the incisor edges. If an attempt is made to take the arrowheads right up to the gingival margin then too great an undercut will be engaged and the wire will be severely flexed when the molar clasps are disengaged and pulled down during removal of the appliance.

A further disadvantage of the Adams' universal clasp is that it suits only those situations where retentive arrowheads are required in groups of two. In situations where this is not the case, e.g. when first molars are already clasped and the operator wishes to clasp the mesial of the second premolars, a problem arises.

The accessory clasp often advised for this situation incorporates a soldered joint where the auxiliary wire joins the bridge of the molar clasp. This represents a potential weakness.

The Single Arrowhead Clasp

In the situation just described, a single arrowhead clasp in 0.8 mm wire placed on the mesiobuccal corner of the upper second premolar is preferable. The increased gauge of the wire makes it robust yet easy to adjust and avoidance of the soldered joint makes construction simpler and lessens the likelihood of breakage. The same simple device makes a good alternative to the single arrowhead version of the universal clasp described for use on the mesial of upper second molars which often gives only indifferent retention. The single arrowhead is simply formed by bending and pinching up the end of a piece of 0.8 mm wire. This can be fitted onto the model in the same way as for a universal clasp, the wire being adapted over the embrasure and the tag finished off palatally. The absence of the bridge makes accurate positioning and adjustment easy at the chairside and the thicker gauge of the wire compensates for any loss of rigidity. The adaptability of single arrowheads makes them very useful for situations where molars do not offer good retention and they can be especially useful in the construction of lower appliances. Ball ended clasps may also be used in these situations. They are of similar design and blanks may be obtained from dental supply companies.

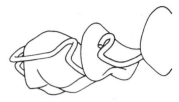

A single arrowhead clasp is contoured over the contact point and provides flexibility and sufficient wire for easy adjustment.

Incisor Clasps

It has already been pointed out that although the Adams' clasp can be used on anterior teeth it is often not ideal in this situation. Various alternative clasps can be used and like the Adams' clasp are constructed in 0.7 mm wire.

The Short Fitted Wire

On proclined incisors this is preferable. The absence of arrowheads means that if the usual method of removal is used there is very little flexion of the clasp during insertion. The wire is a useful guide for the patient who is new to the appliance. It is positioned over the central incisors and the back of the appliance pushed up into place. This locks the labial wire into position giving excellent retention. The same design but with the incorporation of small loops is useful if the incisors are only mildly proclined. The loops fit flush

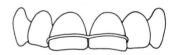

A simple fitted wire gives good retention on proclined incisors.

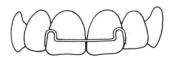

The fitted labial wire with small adjustment loops.

against the labiodistal corners of the central incisors and themselves offer some retention. This clasp stands out less than the universal clasp and is also a better choice where there is a midline space. The close fit of the wire prevents any mesial movement of the teeth under the influence of pressure from the arrowheads.

The Long Fitted Wire

In situations where the lateral incisors bear a good relationship to the centrals it is possible to include these teeth in the clasp. This has the advantage that the wire crosses the lateral/canine embrasure rather than the central/lateral embrasure. The morphology of the teeth makes this easier in most cases and the clasp is also less prone to damage by the lower incisors. This clasp is not kept incisally but lies halfway up the labial face of the incisors where some undercut may more easily be engaged between the teeth. This is important as the greater length of wire renders the clasp more flexible and makes it necessary to engage a deeper undercut. The lateral incisor often tends to escape from this clasp unless the wire is kept well gingivally where it passes round the distal aspect of this tooth. If the relationship between the lateral incisor and canine does not permit this then the small loops provide sufficient wire for this part to be adjusted gingivally when space becomes available.

Where the incisors are severely proclined there is little to gain by contouring this wire around the teeth and a plain wire bow across the incisors with small loops by the laterals offers good retention.

The Long Labial Bow

It is common for a long labial bow to be incorporated into an appliance being used for retraction of canines prior to reduction of an overjet. This is sometimes done in the hope that the labial bow will help to improve anchorage and retention during canine retraction and can subsequently be activated itself to reduce the overjet. Such a hope is usually forlorn as a bow which is flexible enough to carry out tooth movement is too flexible to splint the incisors and so provide 'static' anchorage. Furthermore unless the incisors are severely proclined such a bow is unlikely to offer very much by way of retention.

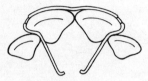

In some cases careful contouring is necessary to take the wire over the contact points.

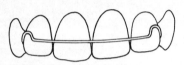

A fitted labial wire designed to control the lateral incisors.

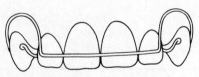

The long labial bow. This contributes little to anchorage or retention.

PASSIVE WIREWORK

It is sometimes necessary to include wire components to prevent unwanted spontaneous drifting of teeth. This particularly applies adjacent to extraction sites and to prevent the relapse of recently moved teeth. These stops may conveniently be constructed in soft 0.7 mm stainless steel wire which, while providing adequate resistance to movement, permits ease of adjustment at the chairside. They should be sited across the appropriate surfaces of the tooth and placed so as not to interfere with nearby planned tooth movements.

Stops Following Extractions

Upper First Molar Extractions

When these teeth have recently been, or are about to be, extracted, stops may be placed mesial to the second molars to prevent their rapid forward drift. Occasionally some movement may be desirable to allow full eruption of the clinical crown for subsequent clasping, in which case mesial drifting may be permitted for some weeks prior to appliance construction. Alternatively the stop may be sited some way mesial to the second molar.

Upper Premolar Extractions

When a premolar has been extracted the first molar will usually be clasped thereby preventing any unwanted movement. The second premolar shows no tendency to drift mesially away from the first molar, so that after first premolar extractions it is unnecessary to provide mesial stops.

Upper Incisor Extractions

These teeth show a great tendency to drift towards extraction sites and therefore appropriate stops are often required to control unwanted movements.

Stops Following Tooth Movement

Any recently moved tooth shows a tendency to relapse towards its former position. Unless the new appliance prevents such movement by reason of base plate design or clasp placement then a passive stop must be provided. The commonest indication occurs following canine retraction and prior to incisor alignment or overjet reduction.

CHAPTER 4

Principles of Design:
Active Components – Springs
and Elastics

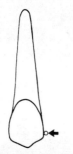

The ideal situation. It is possible to apply the force at almost 90° to the long axis of the tooth.

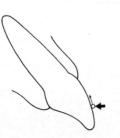

Activation of a labial wire will cause it to move gingivally on proclined incisors.

The active components of removable appliances are those which exert the force which produces tooth movement. Possible active components include springs, screws and elastics. The authors use elastics only infrequently with removable appliances, and screws (which are dealt with in Chapter 5) are restricted to a limited number of situations. Springs constitute without any doubt the majority of active components.

SPRINGS

General Principles

The design and placement of a spring determine the direction in which it will apply its force. Three principles are important with all types of spring:

1. *The force should be delivered at right angles to the long axis of the tooth.* When this principle is met all the force applied to the tooth is used to achieve movement. When it is not met a vertical component of force is produced which will tend to displace the spring. Examples of such displacement may be seen during retraction of a canine with a poorly positioned buccal spring or when a labial bow is activated palatally on proclined incisors.

2. *As far as possible the force should be applied through a surface which is parallel to the long axis of the tooth.* Failure to comply with this will not only cause displacement of the spring but can sometimes produce unwanted intrusion of the tooth. The displacement may be corrected by altering the direction of spring activation so that it is more nearly at right angles to the surface to which it is applied, but this will increase the tendency to intrude the tooth and will produce

26

an increased displacing force on the appliance. An example of this may be seen when an attempt is made to retract a partially erupted canine by activating the spring on the sloping mesial surface of the cusp. It also occurs when an incisor is proclined by spring activation on the sloping surface of the cingulum.

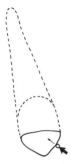

The spring can only be stabilized by incorporating some upward activation which will hinder eruption and displace the appliance.

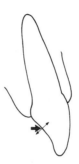

Forward activation of a palatal spring against the sloping lingual surface of an incisor will tend to displace the appliance.

3. *The force should pass through the centre of resistance of the tooth (approximately the centre of the tooth viewed in cross-section).* When this does not occur there will be a tendency for the tooth to rotate. This may frequently be seen when buccally placed canines are retracted by means of finger springs. Buccal springs are preferable in this respect but a closer examination of any cases where rotation has occurred during canine retraction commonly reveals that a slight rotation was present initially. The use of a more complex technique might well have been advisable.

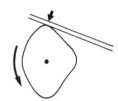

Activation of this palatal spring will tend to rotate the tooth mesio-buccally as it is retracted.

SPRING DESIGNS

Springs for Mesiodistal Movement

The Palatal Finger Spring

This is commonly used to retract a canine after the removal of the first premolar. It can also be used to move any tooth mesially or distally along the arch.

The simplest form of this spring is a straight piece of wire embedded at one end into the acrylic base plate. The usual wire diameter is 0.5 mm or occasionally 0.6 mm. In practice

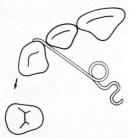

The coil is correctly positioned to apply a force at right angles to the direction of desired movement.

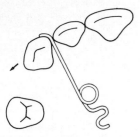

Incorrect coil position is liable to produce unwanted buccal movement.

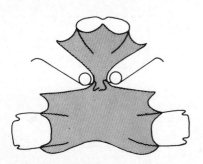

Obvious midline weakness produced by the use of bilateral open springs.

a coil is incorporated near the insertion into the acrylic. This allows an increased length of wire to be accommodated within the confined space and so makes possible the delivery of a light force over a long distance. The coil should be made as large as possible consistent with fitting it into the appliance, say 3 to 4 mm. By convention it is placed so that when activated it is tightened as the appliance is inserted and uncoils as the tooth moves (i.e. the coil is on the side of the wire away from the direction of tooth movement). This has recently been shown to be of little importance.

A coil spring of this design will usually be about 2 cm in length from the point of application to its insertion into the acrylic. The position of the coil is most important as it influences the direction in which the spring works. This will be dealt with more fully in the section on applied design.

Advantages. The spring provides a light pressure and is well tolerated. Several springs can be added if required to retract teeth successively. *Disadvantages.* The palatal finger spring cannot move teeth in a palatal direction. It is thus unsuitable for buccally placed teeth and its use in such circumstances may move a tooth further buccally and tend to produce rotation.

The base plate must not hinder movement of the spring and this can be prevented in the following ways:

Open Spring

The spring is formed on the model and, except for the locking tag, waxed in before the acrylic is added (in the case of heat cured acrylic the spring would have to be plastered in). The appliance is then constructed so that the spring is left free to move and is not covered by acrylic. Its full length is visible in the mouth when the appliance is in place.

Advantages. Cleaning is made very easy and binding of the spring against the acrylic is eliminated. If the spring does become distorted it can be readily adjusted. Wire guards can be incorporated if necessary to limit distortion.
Disadvantages. If identical springs are placed bilaterally the appliance is weakened and the remaining isthmus of acrylic has to be thickened in compensation.

Boxed Spring

This spring is waxed in during construction in a similar manner to the open spring but the wax is kept shallow and the acrylic is extended over it so that the spring is left free to move in a recess on the fitting surface of the base plate.

At first sight it might seem sufficient to make this recess only large enough to permit the spring to move from its original to its intended final position. It must be remembered, however, that during activation a spring must be flexed beyond the position in which it will finally be passive. It is therefore necessary to extend the recess further distally in order to allow activation of the spring during the final stage of tooth movement.

Advantages. The acrylic cover over the spring strengthens the appliance and gives a smoother surface for the tongue.

Disadvantages. Unless waxing in is carried out carefully insufficient space may be left for the spring to move between the acrylic and the mucosa. Alternatively the thickness of the appliance may be unduly increased.

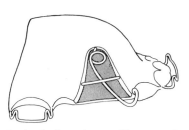

Boxing in the spring provides protection and strengthens the base plate.

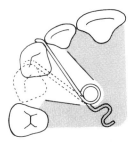

Suggested limits of the recess for a boxed spring to permit access for activation.

Guard Wires

A guard wire may be incorporated to prevent displacement or distortion of a spring during wear. An open spring may have a guard wire placed on the tongue side or may occasionally have wires on each side of it so that in action it slides between the two. A boxed spring may carry a guard wire between itself and the soft tissue of the palate to prevent the spring from becoming distorted away from the acrylic during wear (such distortion, once it has occurred, may be difficult to correct).

In either case the guard, to be of any use, must be placed well down the spring from the coil, but it must not be carried near enough to the path of tooth movement to impede the necessary trimming of the acrylic. It is usually constructed in 0.5 mm wire and made with a slight curve so that it follows the shape of the arch.

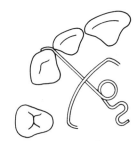

A correctly sited guard wire is a useful accessory.

Advantages. A carefully positioned guard wire can be a definite aid during tooth movement and can limit distortion of the spring. If a broken finger spring has to be replaced the guard wire can hold the new spring in position while the acrylic is cured around its locking tag.

Disadvantages. A wrongly positioned guard wire may be useless or may even hinder tooth movement. It is also easy to leave too little space for the spring between the guard wire and the acrylic.

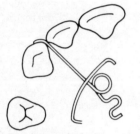

Incorrect, the guard wire is too close to the coil to be effective.

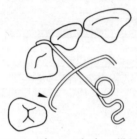

Incorrect, the guard wire will hinder the later stages of canine retraction.

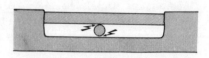

Incorrect, there is insufficient clearance between the guard wire and acrylic to permit free movement of the spring.

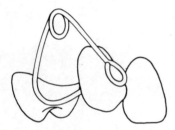

A popular design of buccal canine retractor constructed in 0.7 mm wire.

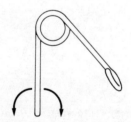

The efficiency of this spring may be reduced by rotation about its insertion into the acrylic.

The Buccal Canine Retractor

The overall shape of this spring can be seen in the figure. It comprises a posterior arm which passes across the line of the arch and up into the sulcus to support a coil from which the anterior arm descends to engage the canine. It is particularly suitable in situations where the canine overlaps the lateral incisor labially. It is usually made in 0.7 mm wire but can also be constructed in 0.5 mm wire with the supporting arm sheathed in 0.5 mm (i.d.) hard stainless steel tubing. Because the spring curves up into the sulcus at over 90° to its insertion into the base plate it tends, during use, to rotate within the acrylic rather like the action of turning a door handle. To prevent this a definite crank must be made to lock the spring into the base plate. It is not sufficient to turn the wire down on to the surface of the model as for an Adams' clasp. Care must be taken to position this crank so that it will not limit the later stages of canine retraction.

If the spring crosses mesial to the second premolar at gingival level it will prevent full retraction of the canine and although this can be corrected at the chairside during the later stages of retraction it is better if the spring is constructed to cross the premolar at the level of the interstitial ridge. For this reason it is helpful to present the technician with a model before extraction and to discourage the habit of cutting the tooth to be extracted off the model. The coil

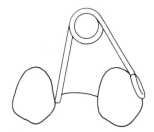

This is an example of a well-proportioned spring but the supporting arm enters the acrylic at gingival level.

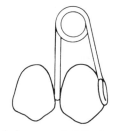

This design prevents full retraction of the canine.

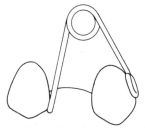

A correctly positioned arm to permit contact between the canine and second premolar.

should be of about 3 mm (i.d.) and placed so that if its position remained constant during movement the anterior arm would swing like a pendulum. In reality the coil will not maintain a constant position because the whole spring flexes in use but nevertheless the above method will give the correct coil position and allow the anterior arm to lie more or less parallel to the mesial surface of the canine and so deliver its force at 90° to the long axis of the tooth. This will avoid displacement of the spring. If the impression is well muscle trimmed it should help the technician to position the coil so that it is not likely to cause trauma to the sulcus and does not conflict with the muscle attachment in this area. It may only be necessary to turn the end of the anterior arm through a right angle toward the mid-line and cut it off to leave a foot of about 2 mm which will engage the mesial edge of the canine. When the spring is activated, however, this foot may tend to slip buccally from the tooth unless the whole spring is swung a little in a palatal direction which may in turn have the unwanted effect of causing trauma to the gingival margin. A better design of foot is made by turning the end of the spring into a loop of about 3 mm dia. which engages the canine securely and rests against the gingival margin rather than sticking into it, see illustration of buccal canine retractor.

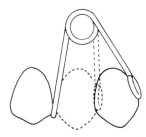

A correctly sited coil with both arms of approximately equal length.

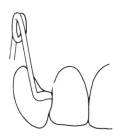

A useful alternative way of engaging the canine.

If the canine is partially erupted a simple foot can be used but can be improved if the end is annealed, flattened to resemble a golfing iron and curved to fit the surface of the canine.

Advantages. The spring offers good control of the canine during distal movement. It prevents unwanted buccal movement and its end can be turned through 90° and used to tuck the canine palatally, if necessary, at the end of retraction. It generally displaces the appliance less than a

31

palatal spring and is usually well accepted by adults because it is frequently unnecessary to use clasping on the anterior teeth.

Disadvantages. The heavy gauge of the wire makes it easy to exert excess pressure on the canine. Unless the spring is properly proportioned and constructed it may be unstable in the vertical plane and difficult to control. It can also cause trauma to the sulcus and is readily distorted.

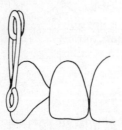

The canine is retracted but still buccally placed. The spring has been modified to correct this.

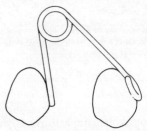

A badly proportioned spring with arms of unequal length and the coil too far distally.

An Alternative Buccal Retraction Spring

An alternative design is shown here. The authors rarely use this spring but it can be particularly useful for buccally placed canines which erupt fairly high up on the buccal surface of the alveolus with a mesial inclination. It is also of particular use with lower appliances. As is the case with the normal buccal spring this spring is constructed in 0.7 mm wire but instead of a coil it merely has a large loop in the sulcus from which the mesial arm of the spring engages onto the canine. The spring can be designed with or without a reversed loop as desired. In either case it is important that the loop should be made sufficiently large to give good flexibility to the spring and that the spring itself should be so shaped that the arm which engages the tooth lies at approximately right angles to the mesial surface.

Advantages. The spring is useful for buccally placed canines and is less likely to traumatize the sulcus. This makes it especially applicable to lower removable appliances.

Disadvantages. Once again the spring tends to be fairly rigid and activation can be difficult to control.

Spring for Buccal Movement

Cranked Palatal Spring 0.5 mm

A palatal finger spring of the type already described can, if angled correctly, be used to move an individual tooth buccally. In most cases a crank is bent into the spring so that during

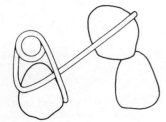

This design may be useful where the sulcus is shallow. In this example a coil has been incorporated.

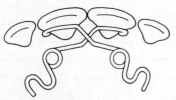

The spring can be used singly or in pairs as in this example.

the later stages of activation it does not contact neighbouring teeth.

Advantages. The spring gives a controllable light force. Its coil and the arm, as far as the crank, derive some protection and stability from the covering of the acrylic. The direction of activation can be varied slightly and the use of two such springs, crossed, can be helpful when two upper incisors have to be proclined.

Disadvantages. The space necessary to incorporate the spring may bring it into conflict with other wirework. It is not suitable for posterior teeth such as premolars which have an almost vertical lingual surface. In this situation the wire tends to catch on the occlusal surface during insertion even with very slight activation.

The Double Cantilever or 'Z' Spring 0.5 mm

This is a variant of the palatal finger spring and is the commonest type in this series. The name is self-explanatory as the spring is bent into the shape of a 'Z' with two coils. It should be constructed with the spring compressed and the presence of two coils makes it possible for the end of the spring delivering the force to be activated in a straight line rather than to move through the arc of a circle.

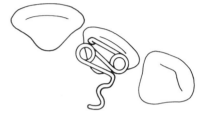

The 'Z' spring may be used singly as in the example or made larger to move two adjacent teeth simultaneously.

Advantages. The spring is compact and may be incorporated on a small tooth such as a lateral incisor even when there is clasping on the centrals and a spring on the canine. A larger spring may be constructed to act on two neighbouring teeth. The force is delivered in a straight line and the spring may be given a slight upward activation which will allow easier insertion and will not trap the spring between the acrylic and the enamel.

Disadvantages. It is less suitable for posterior teeth because, as is the case with the cranked palatal finger spring, it is readily trapped on the occlusal surfaces of the teeth during insertion. If the spring is made very small it can easily produce an excessive force during activation. If the spring is used for more than a slight amount of movement there may be problems with its vertical stability. The reactionary force to this spring from the incisal cingulum tends to displace the anterior part of the appliance. Good anterior retention is therefore essential.

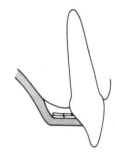

The boxed in 'Z' spring aligned as near as possible at 90° to the long axis of the tooth.

The 'T' Spring 0.5 mm

Again the shape is self-explanatory. Both ends of the wire are embedded into the base plate and the cross piece rests on the palatal surface of the tooth to be moved. The addition of extra bends half way up the spring increases its flexibility and provides spare wire for its extension during tooth movement.

Advantages. The spring is particularly suitable to provide buccal movement of buccal teeth. Its action means that it is less likely to catch on

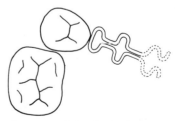

The most useful spring for buccal movement of premolars and canines.

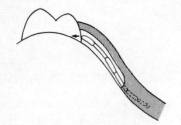

Palatal view of boxed in 'T' spring.

the occlusal surface of such a tooth during insertion. The provision of extra loops extends its range of activation. It occupies only a small space and can be used on a premolar concurrently with other movements such as canine retraction.

Disadvantages. If this spring is used to procline an incisor it will inevitably deliver a strong upward component of force through the cingulum.

All these springs are generally boxed in under the acrylic of the base plate. Skilful construction is necessary if the springs are not to make the acrylic excessively bulky.

Springs for Lingual Movement

Various designs are available, all emerging from the acrylic, crossing the embrasure and passing up towards the sulcus. The type of end is determined by the relationship of an available embrasure and also by the activation and pressure required. These springs must be robust and 0.7 mm wire is generally used.

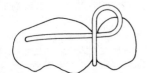

This spring is occasionally used for correction of a buccally displaced molar.

The Molar Spring

Here a reversed loop is used to allow the spring to press on the buccal surface of a buccally placed molar.

The Canine and Premolar Spring

This spring owes its origin to the buccal canine retractor and such a retractor can be adapted to this shape to correct the canine which is outstanding at the end of its retraction. A loop-ended buccal spring lends itself to this design, since the loop provides the available wire to reshape (after softening locally in a flame to anneal the wire). Many types of buccal spring in use do not provide enough wire for this modification.

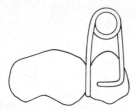

A convenient design of spring for the palatal movement of premolars and canines.

Single Incisor Spring

A further modification of the buccal canine retractor is useful in the correction of an outstanding lateral incisor when a Class II, division 2 type of case is being treated by alignment of the upper arch only. The wire emerges from the acrylic and crosses the mesial surface of the second premolar. It then passes up into the sulcus and forwards over the canine eminence before descending to engage the labial face of the lateral incisor with a flattened loop. It can be incorporated into the same appliance as a palatal finger spring which will be used to correct the canine prior to the

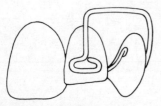

This spring is used for the alignment of a single outstanding incisor.

activation of the incisor spring. Such a design of spring can also be used occasionally to correct a single outstanding central incisor.

Advantages. Remember that buccal springs carry out movements which cannot be achieved with lingual springs. The modification just described to align an outstanding incisor offers more control than can be obtained from a labial bow.

Disadvantages. In common with all buccal springs excessive force, trauma to the sulcus and ease of distortion can provide problems.

Soldered Auxiliary Spring 0.6 mm *Wire or* 0.7 mm *Wire*

An auxiliary spring may be soldered to the bridge of the clasp on the first molar. Two versions are available. The spring can be used to tuck an outstanding canine or pre-molar into line during the final stages of treatment.

Advantages. The spring does not cross the embrasure and so does not compete with other wire work. (As a general principle it is sensible to avoid, wherever possible, placing two wires through a single embrasure.) The spring can be added easily to an existing appliance and if necessary may be cranked to correct an outstanding canine through the loop of the labial bow on a retainer. The length and hence the flexibility of the spring can be controlled by a choice of the appropriate wire size and where necessary by bringing the wire from the distal end of the bridge of the clasp and recurving it forwards. (This may be particularly useful when a second pre-molar has to be moved palatally.)

Disadvantages. A certain level of expertise with solder is required if the spring is to be attached satisfactorily without annealing the wire of the clasp. It is also difficult to add this spring to a clasp which is already carrying a soldered tube for the application of a face bow.

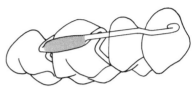
This spring has the advantage that it may be added easily to an existing appliance.

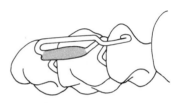
The spring can be recurved to achieve flexibility.

Springs for the Reduction of Overjet and Alignment of Incisors

A wide variety of appliances and springs have been designed to carry out these movements. This is no doubt because of the lack of an ideal spring. Each type has its advantages and disadvantages which may be more or less important to different situations and operators.

Heavy Wire:
The Labial Bow with Small Loops—0.7 mm *Wire*

This is unsuitable for the reduction of anything but the smallest overjet and for squeezing irregular incisors into line. Larger overjets would take a long time to reduce. A very small activation of the bow will produce an excessive force and such force may lead to anchorage loss or to discomfort

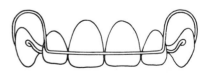
A compromise design of more use on a retainer than on an active appliance.

35

which results in non-wear of the appliance. This type of bow is still widely used, however, and is often found incorporated into an appliance bearing palatal finger springs to retract the canines. No doubt this is done in an attempt to reduce the number of appliances required for a given case. In the authors' opinion such an approach is often a false economy and this type of bow should be used with caution.

Advantages. The placing of offsets into the bow can, in combination with selective trimming of the acrylic, squeeze irregular incisors into line. The rigidity of the bow makes it suitable for modification as a retainer following active treatment.

Disadvantages. Even slight activation of the wire can readily produce excessive pressure and because of this the bow is unsuitable for the reduction of any but the slightest overjet.

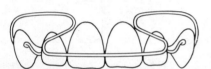

A useful labial bow but not easy to adjust.

Heavy Wire:
The Labial Bow with Large Loops—0.7 mm *Wire*

Loops may be of varying size up to the type incorporated in the bow described by Mills. Although such a bow will give a light pressure over a long distance it is difficult to manufacture and also to adjust. Loops of a less extreme size permit easier adjustment and yet give a light controllable force.

Advantages. It is still possible to put pressure on individual teeth and the bow is useful in retaining the corrected position after tooth movement.

Disadvantages. Skill is required to control the activation of the bow and at the same time prevent the wire from traumatizing the sulcus. The wire tends to slide gingivally up proclined teeth and must therefore be activated occlusally. Sometimes it is difficult to maintain the wire at the right position on the teeth.

An easily activated spring giving a light, controlled force.

Light Wire:
The Roberts' Retractor

The retractor described by Roberts is shown. It is constructed in 0.5 mm wire but the buccal arms are sheathed from the coil into the acrylic with 0.5 mm (i.d.) hard stainless steel tubing to provide added strength.

Advantage. This spring produces a light force and is easily adjustable. Because it swings downwards and backwards during use it does not tend to slide gingivally up proclined incisors and it is well tolerated.

Disadvantages. If the supporting arms are not correctly positioned the sulcus may be traumatized. In the event of breakage major reconstruction will be necessary.

Light Wire:
The Apron Spring

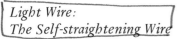

The shape of this spring is almost self-explanatory. It is constructed in 0.5 mm wire and is wound on to a split high labial bow in 0.9 mm wire.

Advantages. Its action is similar to the Roberts' retractor and the same advantages apply. In the event of breakage it is simpler to repair and an experienced operator can replace the light wire at the chairside.

Disadvantages. The spring is rather more likely than the Roberts' retractor to cause trauma to the sulcus and it must be carefully adjusted and maintained.

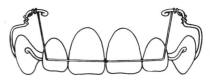

A light wire spring wound onto heavy supporting arms.

Light Wire:
The Self-straightening Wire

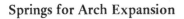

The basis of this spring is a labial bow in 0.7 mm wire incorporating medium adjustment loops. A light wire is wound on to the corner of one of these loops and its end hooked to the other side of the labial wire. The retraction force is provided by the tendency of the light wire to straighten itself across the arc formed by the heavy labial bow. It is best to use a pair of these springs crossing in the midline to avoid any tendency to flatten one side of the arch anteriorly.

Advantages. The overjet can be reduced using a light wire which gives a light force. Subsequently the heavy labial bow can be adjusted into contact with the teeth to provide retention. Because of the support given by the heavy wire vertical stability of the light wire is good.

Disadvantages. It can be difficult to control the degree of activation which is largely 'built in' by the technician. If the spring is not well constructed it is easy to find that it does not slide freely and that binding occurs. Unless bilateral wires are used and carefully controlled it is easy to produce flattening of the arch anteriorly. Trauma to the lip may occur as the incisors move back between adjustments and the heavy wire is left prominent.

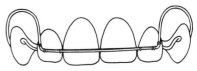

Another method using a light wire auxilliary.

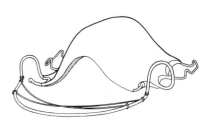

Two fine wires are used to maintain arch symmetry.

Springs for Arch Expansion

The Coffin Spring

In cases where lateral expansion of the upper arch is required this spring may provide a suitable alternative to the use of a screw. The indications for upper arch expansion are discussed in Chapter 5.

The Coffin spring is constructed from 1.25 mm wire and made to the design shown. When constructing an appliance incorporating this spring the following points are important:

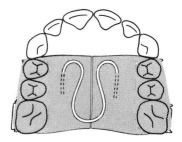

An appliance using a Coffin spring to provide bilateral expansion.

37

a. Whenever arch expansion is being carried out good retention is vital. Four clasps should be provided.

b. To permit the full range of activation the anterior bends must not be incorporated into the acrylic.

c. To improve patient acceptance the spring should be sited as high as possible in the palatal vault.

Activation. This can be carried out by expanding the appliance manually or by reducing the curvature of the bends by use of pliers. To achieve parallel opening all the bends must be adjusted. Activation of the anterior bends or the main posterior curve will produce posterior or anterior expansion respectively.

Measurements. Small bur marks may be made anteriorly and posteriorly on each side of the palate. These provide points of reference for dividers and enable the operator to assess arch expansion.

Advantages. The spring is cheap by comparison with a screw and easier for the patient to keep clean. It permits non-parallel expansion when this is required and the patient does not have to adjust the appliance. It can also provide more rapid movement than can be provided by a screw.

Disadvantages. Correct construction demands a high degree of skill from the technician. Excellent retention is necessary to ensure that the appliance does not displace. It can also easily be over-activated.

ELASTIC TRACTION

Most fixed appliance techniques commonly use elastics to provide intermaxillary and intramaxillary traction.

In removable appliance treatment elastics are employed only rarely.

Intermaxillary Traction

It is possible to use traction from hooks on a removable appliance to a fixed or removable appliance in the opposing jaw. This is an inconvenient and inefficient procedure and cases requiring such an approach are usually unsuited to treatment with removable appliances.

Intramaxillary Traction

The only common use of elastic traction is as a way of moving upper incisors palatally to reduce an overjet. Latex elastics may be obtained in various sizes from orthodontic supply companies.

An elastic of suitable size is attached from a buccal hook placed by each upper canine. The height of the hook must be such that the elastic will rest about half way up the labial faces of the upper incisors. The elastic must be changed every few days.

Advantages. 1. The elastic is almost invisible and this is welcomed by a patient who is concerned by the visibility of the appliance.

2. If an anterior wire is being used to reduce an overjet and is broken during use it may be possible to reshape the ends into hooks and attach an elastic. Treatment can then continue without delay.

Disadvantages. 1. It is impossible to control the force on an individual tooth by comparison with a labial wire which may be contoured. This prevents the correction of local irregularities.

2. There is often a tendency to flatten the arch.

3. The elastic can easily slide upwards and cause trauma to the gingival margin.

4. In contrast to a wire an elastic cannot be passified. There is no way of retaining the corrected tooth position.

CHAPTER 5

Principles of Design: Screws

When an appliance is inserted into the mouth any spring which is active must flex in order to seat in the correct position against the tooth which is to be moved. Once in place it will deliver a continuous light force which will decrease gradually over several weeks as the tooth moves.

The action of an orthodontic screw is very different. Various types of small screws have been used to move individual teeth buccally but they do not seem to offer any advantages over a suitable design of spring. An orthodontic screw does not usually contact the teeth and is embedded at both ends into the acrylic which is subsequently split with a saw. Activation is achieved by turning the screw so that the two sections of the acrylic are moved apart and the appliance, which is still rigid, will not fit completely passively. As it is pushed into position the acrylic or the wirework will deliver force to the teeth. A slight amount of adaptive movement can be accommodated by the periodontal membrane and bony adaptation subsequently occurs. If the screw is over activated the appliance cannot be fully seated.

SCREW DESIGNS

Screws are produced by a number of manufacturers and a wide range of sizes and types is available.

A typical design has a central threaded screw, each end of which engages into a small metal or plastic block. One of these blocks carries two guide wires which lie parallel to the screw and pass through holes in the opposing block. The centre of the screw is enlarged into a small boss in which four radially positioned holes are visible. A small wire key is supplied and may be inserted into one of these holes and

 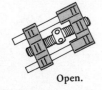

Closed.   Open.

A typical orthodontic screw.

turned like a capstan through 90° until it touches the guide. For further activation the procedure must be repeated with the key inserted into the next hole.

Until recently it was necessary for the technician to box in the central portion of the screw with plaster (or with wax if a cold cure system was being used) so that the acrylic did not encroach on to the moving parts and prevent activation. Most modern patterns of screw are supplied with a soft plastic tag covering the central portion. The tag provides a convenient way of holding the screw in place during appliance construction and is torn off after processing. Screws are available in two forms. In one type the threaded pin and guides project beyond the blocks when the screw is closed. In the other the metal or plastic coverage is extended so that no projections are visible. Either type can be cured in the closed position and then opened but an attempt to cure the former sort in the open position and close it subsequently will be unsuccessful. The acrylic behind the blocks will not permit the screw to project beyond the metal as it is turned.

A number of points must be borne in mind when considering whether to use a screw or spring for a particular task.

Bulk

Despite the decreasing size of modern orthodontic screws an appliance carrying a screw still has to be considerably thicker than one without. Unless particular care is taken it is easy during the construction to thicken the entire vault of the palate even when the screw is situated on one side.

Patient Co-operation

We have pointed out that unlike a spring a screw can only be activated to give a small amount of movement over the course of a few days. For this reason it is not adequate for the operator to adjust the appliance monthly. Regular very slight activation must be provided and the screw must usually be turned by the patient through a quarter of a revolution once or twice weekly. If it is turned less frequently progress will be very slow. If it is turned more frequently then the fit may gradually deteriorate. More reliance has to be placed on the patient and it is doubly important to make sure that he or she knows exactly what is to be done and can demonstrate how to turn the screw successfully before leaving the surgery.

The screw should always be turned from the polished side of the appliance and if it is not ready made with an arrow to indicate the direction of turning, then the technician should be asked to place such a mark nearby in the acrylic.

Clasping

When using a screw it is possible to move teeth which are to be clasped. This can be extremely useful when there is a shortage of claspable teeth. The fact that the force is delivered to the teeth by the acrylic or the wirework means that screws are especially suitable where groups of teeth must be moved.

SCREW POSITIONING

It has been stressed that it is important to position the loops of finger springs accurately but we have pointed out that some degree of compensatory adjustment can be carried out during tooth movement with such a spring. The direction of action of a screw can only be varied by cutting out the screw and re-curing it. It is therefore most important that the screw is accurately positioned in three dimensions during construction. For example:

(1) As a molar tooth is pushed distally it will move along the curve of Spee rather like the sweep of a pendulum. When a screw is being used to provide this distal movement it must be angled so that activation moves the molar clasp upwards and backwards or the clasp and acrylic will disengage from the tooth as activation proceeds.

2. In the same example of distal movement of a molar, the screw must be positioned so that the arch is widened as the

Screw position — alignment relative to the curve of Spee.

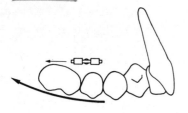

Incorrect, activation of the screw will disengage the clasp from the molar as it moves distally.

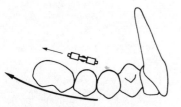

Correct, the fit of the appliance should be maintained as the molar moves distally.

Screw position — alignment relative to arch form.

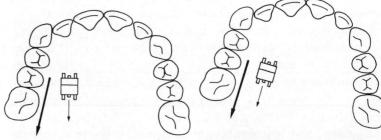

Incorrect, the molar may drop into crossbite as it moves distally.

Correct, the screw is aligned parallel to the buccal segment and will maintain the upper arch form.

molar moves distally and thus maintains a correct bucco-lingual relationship with the lower teeth.

(3) Where a screw is being used to provide arch expansion it will usually be positioned in the midline where it fits easily in a horizontal position. If one or two neighbouring buccal teeth are to be pushed buccally with such a screw then the screw would usually be positioned to one side of the arch and it is tempting to align it parallel to the palatal mucosa rather than horizontally. This would mean that instead of moving the teeth buccally the screw merely disengages the acrylic from them.

Wherever possible the authors generally prefer to use springs rather than screws. For some specific tasks, however, screws can be extremely useful.

Screw position — alignment relative to the palatal vault.

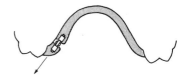

Incorrect, activation of the screw will not move this molar buccally but will merely allow the acrylic to disengage.

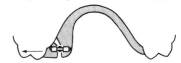

Correct, in this position the screw will produce buccal movement but will inevitably make the appliance much bulkier.

CLINICAL INDICATIONS

Expansion

It is sometimes necessary to increase the width of the upper arch to cure a unilateral crossbite. If this is contemplated it is important that a lateral mandibular displacement can be demonstrated when the patient closes. The absence of a

Correction of unilateral crossbite.

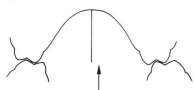

The apparent asymmetry is produced by a lateral displacement of the mandible.

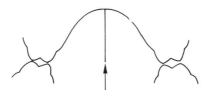

With the mandible in centric relationship the symmetry of the condition is revealed. The teeth occlude cusp to cusp.

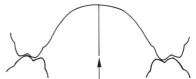

Expansion of the arch width allows a normal bucco-lingual occlusion of the teeth on each side without deviation of the mandible.

lateral displacement means that a true asymmetry is present, either in the form of a local distortion of the alveolus involving a small number of teeth or because of an underlying asymmetry of the face and jaws. Unless the movement of one or two individual teeth will correct the condition it will usually be necessary to consider correlated treatment of both arches.

The presence of a displacement accounts for the apparent asymmetry and shows that the underlying condition is really symmetrical and is due to a slight discrepancy in arch widths

A suitable appliance design for the correction of a unilateral crossbite.

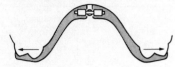

The coronal view.

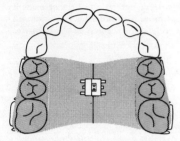

The occlusal view. Four clasps are advisable and posterior bite planes are required. It is not necessary to extend the appliance around the anterior teeth unless movement of these teeth is also desired.

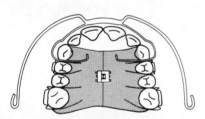

A variety of En-Masse appliance. In this example the face bow is an integral part of the appliance. Molar capping is not required since expansion merely maintains a normal buccal relationship during distal movement.

which can be corrected by treatment of the upper arch alone.

Symmetrical widening of the upper arch can be produced by an upper removable appliance and a suitable design would incorporate four clasps, perhaps on first molars and premolars, with a screw placed horizontally in the mid-line of the palate. The acrylic can be cut back from the incisors (unless an instanding tooth is to be moved as part of the treatment) and the provision of shallow posterior bite planes helps to relieve cuspal interlock and so prevent any secondary widening of the lower arch.

In the case of a bilateral crossbite the discrepancy between the arch widths is much greater than in the case of a unilateral condition. Although the condition is symmetrical treatment with a simple removable appliance is usually inadequate and correlated treatment of both arches would be necessary.

A bilateral crossbite. Although the condition is symmetrical the amount of tooth movement required for correction is much greater than in the unilateral condition.

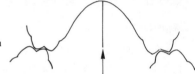

Lateral expansion may also be required as a complementary movement when buccal teeth are being moved distally with extra oral traction. A similar clasping plan would be suitable but posterior bite planes would usually not be necessary.

The extra oral traction could be applied via a detachable face bow to tubes soldered on to molar clasps or alternatively the inner arch of the face bow can be incorporated into the acrylic in the same way as a labial bow. This is frequently known as an 'En-Masse' appliance. In this form it is one of the few removable appliances which does not have to be worn full-time.

Distal Movement

In the previous example the screw was only being used to provide expansion as the extra oral traction provided the distal movement.

An alternative way of moving molars distally is by means of a similar appliance but carrying bilateral screws which will deliver the distal force to the molars. Careful positioning of the screws will be necessary in accordance with the advice given earlier in this chapter. This design has no advantage over the previous one except where different amounts of distal movement are required on each side of the mouth. A version with a screw only on one side is particularly useful when, for example, one upper canine is crowded buccally. In such a situation it may be adequate to clasp the first molars, the first premolar on the other side, and the incisors and to hope that as the screw is turned (again with extra oral force applied via tubes on the molar clasps) the irregularity will improve. If there is any doubt, however, it is better to do this as a two stage procedure beginning once again with four clasps and with the screw opposite the second premolar and going on to a second appliance (still with extra oral support) using finger springs to move the premolars back into the space produced and allow the canine to align.

It is sometimes argued that it is mechanically better to apply the extra oral support to the front part of the appliance rather than to the clasp on the tooth being moved distally. When it is understood that turning the screw tends to push the anterior teeth forwards and the first molar backwards it can readily be seen that the extra oral force is effective when applied to either part of the appliance. It will only be necessary to adjust the loop stop on the inner arch of the face bow to make sure that a firm contact with the molar tube is maintained as movement progresses (see Chapter 10).

Class III Cases

In mild Class III malocclusions with a slight amount of upper arch crowding it is often advisable to avoid upper extractions and use antero-posterior expansion to accommodate the teeth into the arch. The use of extra oral traction alone may tend to worsen the incisor relationship. The use of a removable appliance alone may only achieve alignment by producing an increased and unstable overjet. The use of the appliance just described, with bilateral screws can allow the anterior teeth to be held forwards while the posteriors are moved distally.

CLINICAL MANAGEMENT

When a screw is to be used it is always important to provide very adequate retention. It is safest to be 'slow and sure' and generally the patient should begin by turning the screw a quarter of a revolution once a week. It is sensible to pick a particular day and time when the screw should be turned.

Unilateral creation of space. Retention and efficiency of the appliance will usually be improved if this is carried out as a two stage procedure:

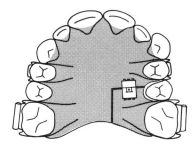

Distal movement of the first molar.

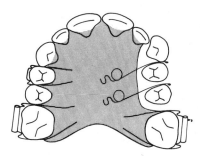

Collection of space in the canine area.

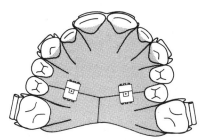

Creation of space bilaterally. This appliance may be very useful where space must be created in an occlusion which tends towards Class III. The anterior teeth are supported forwards as space is made.

Provided that there are the correct number of turns on the screw at the next visit and that the appliance is a good fit, it is possible to increase the turning to two occasions per week at 3 and 4 day intervals. To avoid doubt it is sensible to write down these instructions for the patient. If an appliance with a screw is left out of the mouth relapse can readily occur so that within a few days the appliance can no longer be fitted. For this reason the patient should be instructed to contact the practice immediately in the event of trouble and if this is impossible then to reverse the screw for a few turns until it can be refitted.

Rate of Movement

A typical modern screw has up to forty quarter turns and will open at the rate of 0.2 mm per quarter turn. It follows that an appliance which is correctly adjusted once per week will provide space at the rate of rather less than 1 mm per month.

Fischer Schwartz.
A−D −Vyci

A = Delfyre 4,3mn
dvžice 12,mm

B− Deb − 3mm
Duž 11 mm

Tip A je moguče pričvrti 2u 6,4 mm
360° ohet ⇒ 0,64 mm   10 čitav oheta uluznio
1/4 oheta ⇒ 0,16 mm.   ili 40 × 1/4 oheta.

CHAPTER 6

Treatment Planning
and Applied Design

When a removable appliance is required, the operator has the
opportunity to design a tool specifically suited to the task in
hand. If he is wise he will make full use of this opportunity.
It is true that poor construction may render a good design
useless but not even the most beautiful workmanship will
overcome basic flaws in planning.

It goes without saying that the task of designing belongs
to the operator. No one else will witness so closely the
successes and failures of treatment and be able to modify
future appliance designs in the light of past experience.

Sadly, many dentists are ignorant of appliance design, and
the technician is all too frequently given instructions such as
'please make appliance to retract upper canines'. He will
usually try to do his best and the result will often be usable,
but this sort of arrangement is unfair to all involved. The
patient receives inferior treatment. An operator who is not
in control of the situation can too readily blame the technician, the appliance, or the patient for lack of progress. The
technician, when he is not being blamed, may continue with
his designs in total ignorance of their unfortunate clinical
results.

It is appropriate at this point to mention the personal
relationship between the technician and the dental surgeon.
Ideally the laboratory should be close to the clinical area.
It is then easy for the technician to come to the chairside
and see particular problems. The operator also has access to
the laboratory to give advice and to comment on appliances
while they are under construction. Repairs and modifications
are more easily carried out.

Unfortunately, such an arrangement is often impossible.

Sometimes a local laboratory will collect and deliver work but in many cases impressions are posted to a technician many miles away who may never have met the dental surgeon face to face. In these circumstances great care must be taken that impressions are kept at the correct humidity in sealable plastic bags and that they are well wrapped and protected during transit. It is doubly important that every attempt is made to avoid errors and misunderstandings.

GENERAL PLANNING

At the time of the initial diagnosis and treatment planning the necessary space will have been assessed in relation to the task in hand. Nevertheless, the assessment of space and the control of anchorage are so important that it is wise to check space carefully when planning practical treatment.

Molar Occlusion

In assessing space requirements it must be appreciated that the antero-posterior relationship of the upper and lower molar teeth must be considered. A normal or Class I molar relation is defined when the mesio-buccal cusp of the upper first molar occludes in the buccal groove of the lower first molar. Variations from the normal are described as the displacement of the upper tooth mesially or distally in terms of units.

A unit is usually understood to mean one cusp width mesio-distally; thus molars are two units while canines and premolars are one. Clearly this is only an approximation as the various single unit teeth are not precisely the same size.

A full Class II molar relationship exists where the mesio-buccal cusp of the upper molar occludes in advance of the lower molar, that is, in the groove between the second premolar and the molar.

A half unit Class II molar relationship exists where the upper and lower first molar teeth occlude cusp to cusp, in other words lying mid-way between Class I and a full unit Class II.

A Class III molar relationship exists when the mesio-buccal cusp of the upper first molar occludes distal to the lower molar tooth, and in the groove between first and second molars. Such an occlusion is only found in the small proportion of Class III malocclusions which are most severe.

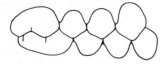

A Class I relationship of buccal teeth.

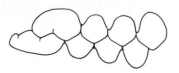

A Class II relationship of buccal teeth.

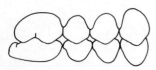

A half unit Class III relationship of buccal teeth.

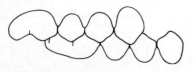

A Class III relationship of buccal teeth.

48

A lesser degree of Class III occlusion is much more likely to be found, and as in the Class II example, lies part-way between normal occlusion and true or full Class III.

Canine Relation

The occlusion of the upper and lower permanent canines may be defined in a similar manner to that of the molars. A Class I relation is when the upper canine occludes distal to the lower and a Class II being when the upper canine occludes mesial to the lower. Half unit Class II canine relationships may be present. If so then the upper canine is often buccally displaced to some extent. Because of the degree of vertical overlap of the canines then in the partial Class II occlusion the upper tooth is pushed labially by the buccal prominence of the lower tooth.

Centre Lines

The relation of the upper and lower centre lines to one another may be of importance, not for intrinsic aesthetic reasons but rather because of the influence it may have on the occlusion of the canines and posterior teeth. This in turn may complicate space assessment.

Lower Incisor Position

When more complex fixed appliance techniques are in use it is common for the antero-posterior position of the lower incisors to be adjusted intentionally. With a removable appliance this is seldom attempted and, although incisor imbrication will often align spontaneously when space is made, the average antero-posterior position of the lower incisors may nevertheless be regarded as a fixed point. This can be extremely useful in planning upper arch treatment.

Space Assessment

Let us take as an example a mild Class II, division 1 malocclusion in which the upper incisors are proclined and the lower labial segment is not crowded.

The upper canines should be visualized as if they had been moved into a Class I relationship with the lowers. This position can then be compared either to the existing spacing or to that which the proposed extractions will produce.

If the lower incisors are imbricated assessment is made

Space assessment.

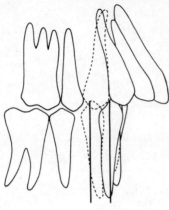

Where there is lower incisor crowding the lower canine will be mesially positioned. Before upper space requirements can be assessed by the previous method it is necessary to imagine the lower canine in its correct position. In this example more upper space will be required than can be provided by the removal of a first premolar.

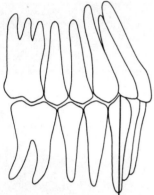

When overjet and overbite are normal the upper canine should have a Class I relationship to the lower arch.

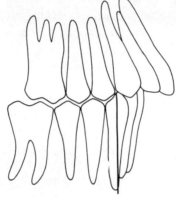

In a Class II, division 1 occlusion the upper canine will be in a forward position.

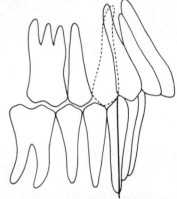

The canine is mentally repositioned into the space which the removal of the first premolar would provide. In this example an upper premolar extraction will be just sufficient provided that no space at all is lost.

more difficult because the lower canines will be mesially placed. It is necessary to re-position the lower canines mentally before making an assessment by the previous method. This can be simplified by marking the corrected position of the lower canines on the study model with a pencil.

Overbite

There is an intimate relationship between overbite and overjet. If a degree of increased overbite is to be accepted (perhaps in a Class II, division 2 type of malocclusion which is to be treated merely by alignment of the outstanding upper lateral incisors) a Class I relationship of the canines will not exist at the end of treatment. Assessment by the previous method is misleading and it is better to assess space by

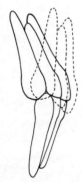

Although overjet may be normal an increase in overbite means that the canine relationship will tend towards Class II.

starting from the upper central incisors and calculating the amount of distal movement of the canines necessary to allow the lateral incisors to be moved into alignment.

Careful examination of the occlusion and the use of the above methods should reveal whether the proposed course of treatment will leave excess space, will give just sufficient space, or whether anchorage reinforcement or complete replanning will be necessary.

THE OVERALL PLAN

Before designing individual appliances it is sensible to work out all the required tooth movements and to have some idea of how these will be carried out. A common fault is to attempt too many tooth movements with one appliance. This may prove a false economy for a number of reasons:

1. *Clasping.* An inadequate number of teeth may be left for clasping. Retention will be poor and it is likely to worsen as treatment proceeds.

2. *Complexity.* It becomes increasingly likely that individual components will interfere with one another. Insertion becomes very difficult and the chance of the appliance being wrongly inserted increases.

3. *Breakage.* The appliance will need to be worn for a longer period of time so that breakages are more likely to be a problem and it may be necessary to reconstruct the appliance completely.

Only very minor courses of treatment can be completed with a single appliance. Commonly two appliances are necessary. In severe cases, or where a special retainer is desirable, three may be required. A case appearing to need more than this should probably be treated by a more sophisticated technique.

The individual tooth movements can be divided among the proposed appliances in such a way that the components on each appliance are compatible, and that adequate retention can be provided for each stage. If anchorage must be reinforced then extra oral traction should be incorporated attached to molar bands; to tubes on molar clasps; or anteriorly to loops or hooks. Retention must be modified if necessary, to facilitate this.

51

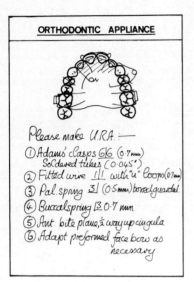

ORTHODONTIC APPLIANCE

Please make U.R.A.:—
① Adams' clasps 6|6 (0.7mm)
   Soldered tubes (0.045")
② Fitted wire 1|1 with "u" loops (0.7mm)
③ Pal. spring 3| (0.5mm) boxed guarded.
④ Buccal spring |3 0.7 mm
⑤ Ant. bite plane, ½ way up cingula
⑥ Adapt preformed face bow as
                              necessary.

A typical appliance diagram with instructions for the technician.

Appliance Planning

The importance of clear concise directions to the technician has been stressed. Full instructions, including wire sizes, should be written legibly for each appliance and a drawing on an idealized arch diagram, is often of great help. A more economic alternative where a printed laboratory sheet is not available is to obtain a rubber stamp representing the upper and lower dental arches. This may be used on a technician's order form where a diagram is not available. Such stamps are often used by those designing partial dentures.

It is sensible to adopt the habit of describing the appliance in a set order so that points are not overlooked. A suitable plan would deal with the components in order as follows:

1. Retention;
2. Passive wirework;
3. Active components;
4. Acrylic modifications;
5. Extra oral components.

We will consider the relevant components in the same order:

Retention

Where possible Adams' clasps on first molars generally make a good basis for retention. Some retention anteriorly will stabilize the appliance. During canine retraction a clasp on both central incisors is usually most suitable and its design will depend upon the degree of incisor proclination which exists. Irregularity of the incisors may mean that it is easier to clasp a single central, a central and lateral, or even two lateral incisors. If the anterior teeth are not suitable for clasping then mesial arrowheads on second premolars will provide some added retention. If the incisors are to be moved then they cannot be clasped. When proclined incisors are being retracted the labial spring will itself help with retention. If necessary Adams' clasps can be used on canines.

During proclination of incisors a clasp on a canine or premolar helps to resist the displacing effect of the spring and in a younger patient a deciduous first molar or canine can be clasped in 0.6 mm wire with good effect.

If first molars have been lost anterior clasping becomes doubly important. The second molars are smaller teeth with a more conical shape. Retention is usually inferior and as the length of the appliance is increased it is much more likely to displace. If the first molars are of poor quality and must be lost it is sometimes more sensible to preserve them temporarily so that they can be used for clasping, e.g. while an instanding upper incisor is moved over the bite. Extraction can be carried out after this correction. Considerable improvisation in design is possible and, for example, a double Adams' clasp on two adjacent premolars will sometimes provide good retention.

Passive Wirework

It is important to prevent unwanted spontaneous tooth movements. For example, it may be necessary to place wire stops on a space maintainer to prevent neighbouring teeth from encroaching into a space while a tooth erupts. It is also usually necessary to place stops mesially to retracted upper canines to prevent the forward relapse of these teeth while an overjet is being reduced.

If unwanted rotation of a canine has occurred during its retraction then the stop on the subsequent appliance should not fit around the tooth but should merely lie across the mesial surface and the acrylic can be trimmed away so that some rotational relapse can occur. The stop should cross the canine on the mesial slope and not at the gingival margin so that the later stages of overjet reduction are not hindered.

Active Wirework

Canine retraction—choice of springs. Remember that there is no need to make the appliance symmetrical and that each side should be designed to suit the problem in that quadrant. Palatal finger springs should be used unless the canine is buccally placed. They are constructed of wire of a thinner diameter than is possible with the buccal spring, and are consequently more flexible. Such flexibility permits the application of a gentle force over a greater distance and will allow longer intervals between adjustments. Coil position is important as it influences the effect of the spring. It is a common mistake to site the palatal coil too far distally and so tend to move the canine buccally as it is retracted. It is wise, therefore, to draw the coil carefully on the design, and if its position is very critical, to make a note bringing this to the technician's attention. Remember that if a buccal canine spring is being used it is not possible to retract the first premolar and canine on the same appliance. If space is

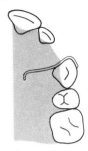

It is not sensible to retain unwanted tooth movements. In this example the canine has rotated slightly during retraction.

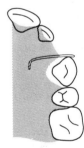

Incorrect, on the second appliance the acrylic and the shaped canine stop form an effective splint to retain the rotation.

Correct, a one-point contact of the stop combined with trimming of the acrylic may permit some spontaneous improvement.

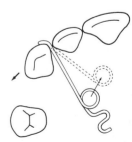

The effect of spring position. The palatal spring shown will move the canine buccally during retraction. The position shown by the dotted line is to be prefered.

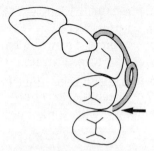

The buccal canine retractor has the disadvantage that because it crosses the arch it can only be used where space has been created immediately distal to the canine.

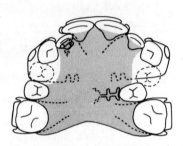

An instanding lateral incisor or premolar can be corrected on the same appliance which is being used to retract the canine. The need to accommodate a crowded premolar may mean that the tooth to be extracted must be cut off the arch and the spring positioned across the extraction space.

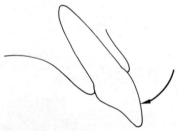

When proclined incisors are to be moved palatally a spring such as the Roberts' retractor is preferred. This swings through the arc of a circle and does not displace itself gingivally.

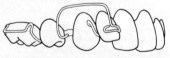

A buccal spring of this design combines well with a palatal spring when an outstanding incisor is to be corrected.

important make sure that the technician does not take the wire of the buccal spring through the extraction space, but keeps it at the level of the marginal ridge.

Concurrent movements. Certain minor movements can be conveniently carried out on the appliance being used for canine retraction. A 'Z' spring can be incorporated to push an instanding lateral incisor labially as space becomes available. A 'T' spring can be incorporated to push an instanding upper second premolar buccally. If space is required for a central incisor then a finger spring can be incorporated on the lateral incisor to take this tooth back in succession to the canine.

Labial springs. A number of springs are available for overjet reduction or incisor alignment. Remember that a large overjet will require light pressure and that heavy wires are only suitable for reducing slight overjets or dealing with imbrication. On severely proclined teeth a spring which swings downwards and backwards such as the Apron spring or Roberts' retractor has an advantage in that it does not slide gingivally. An individually outstanding incisor may be best corrected with a single buccal spring, this will combine very well with a palatal spring which can be used to make space for the correction.

Concurrent movements. Buccally placed teeth can be moved into line during or after overjet reduction by the use of auxiliary springs soldered to the clasp, or springs which cross the embrasure.

54

Acrylic Base Plate

Modification to the acrylic base plate may be necessary to provide anterior or posterior bite planes.

The anterior bite plane. An anterior bite plane is usually required to reduce an increased overbite during the first stage of the treatment of a Class II, division 1 malocclusion, so that subsequent full overjet reduction is possible. It can also be used to provide temporary bite propping to aid the correction of lingually occluding teeth. If an anterior bite plane is required it is sensible to give the technician some indication of its depth by referring to a point on the model which will still be visible when the bite plane is constructed, e.g. 'half-way up the incisor cingula'. It is also sensible, particularly in the case of the severe overjet, to give some indication of how far palatally the bite plane should be taken, perhaps by reference to an imaginary line across the upper canines. The alternative would be to indicate by a drawing on the laboratory card. This will avoid the annoying experience of finding that the lower incisors miss the bite plane altogether. It is important to remember that a bite plane is necessary not only for active reduction of the overbite but also to maintain the reduced overbite. All subsequent appliances must, therefore, carry a bite plane to maintain the ground gained by the first active appliance.

The posterior bite plane. Posterior bite planes are used to aid the correction of bucco-lingual anomalies. The commonest indication is in the treatment of a unilateral posterior crossbite. Rarely it may be used to aid the correction of a reversed incisor overjet where the overbite is much increased.

When posterior bite planes are required it is ideal to let the technician have a lower model. If this is not possible then it should be stressed that the bite planes must be kept shallow particularly at their posterior borders. Unless this is made clear then almost invariably a lot of chairside trimming will be required.

Other modifications to base plate. Time may be saved by having other modifications of the acrylic carried out during construction, e.g. the appliance can be cut away from an outstanding canine or from an erupting premolar. When bite opening is not required then it may not be necessary to extend the acrylic forward to the palatal surfaces of the upper incisors, and this should be made clear to the technician.

Extra Oral Traction

The most secure method of applying extra oral traction to a removable appliance is to insert a face bow in tubes attached to first molar bands. Clips will have to be specified to attach the removable appliance over these tubes. Alternatively the face bow may be applied direct to the appliance, usually by means of tubes which the technician must solder to the bridges of upper first molar clasps. Tube diameter must be specified to suit the wire gauge of the face bow. It is possible to attach a shortened face bow to clasps on other teeth, such as first pre-molars, but this is less satisfactory because retention is often not as good. The use of high pull headgear attached to the anterior part of the appliance is often possible but the necessary hooks or loops must be provided and it is a good idea to make a separate careful drawing of these for the technician.

Whichever method of attaching extra oral traction is selected a suitable face bow will be required. This may be constructed by the technician for each case or, alternatively, selected by the clinician from the stock of factory made preformed face bows. The second alternative is to be preferred because of the superior strength and for reasons of economy. Preformed face bows can readily be cleaned, sterilized and returned to stock for future use.

CONCLUSION

If, after all this, the appliance is manufactured in an unsatisfactory way it is well worthwhile going to some trouble to see the technician, explain to him the problems and the reason for the design and hear his comments. If a specimen appliance can be borrowed from a colleague, it will help to illustrate what is required. It is, of course, a great advantage if the orthodontist himself is able to construct the various components of an appliance and thus show exactly what sort of device he requires.

CHAPTER 7

Lower Removable Appliances

It is often thought that removable appliance treatment must be limited to those cases which require appliances only in the upper arch and where the lower arch either requires no treatment or where extractions alone will allow spontaneous improvement to occur.

This is not entirely true. A combination of an upper removable appliance with a lower fixed appliance is possible (see Chapter 11) and it is also possible to use removable appliances in the lower arch.

Lower removable appliances are commonly held to be very poorly tolerated. It is certainly true that support is poor by comparison with upper appliances which take advantage of the palatal mucosa. Despite this a well made lower appliance designed to carry out limited simple movements will usually be well tolerated and can provide a useful extension to the range of treatment which can be undertaken.

The concurrent wear of upper and lower removable appliances is possible but involves the acceptance of a large bulk of acrylic in the mouth. This combination is therefore better avoided but can be used in selected cases for patients who have proved their ability to co-operate well.

A lower removable appliance can be used where the upper arch is being treated with a fixed appliance or where upper arch treatment is not being carried out simultaneously. The ease with which bite planes may be added makes lower appliances useful to facilitate slight tooth movements in either arch which would otherwise be prevented by the occlusion.

Problems of Construction

Extension

One of the commonest faults with lower appliances is over extension of the acrylic. If the acrylic is extended lingually,

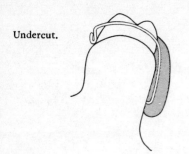

Undercut.

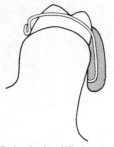

Incorrect, extension of the acrylic into lingual undercut can make the appliance impossible to insert.

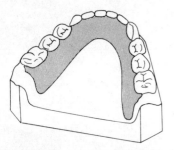

Correct, fitting is simplified and any necessary trimming will not loosen the clasp wire.

The base plate consists of a 'U' shaped strip of acrylic. This restricts the range of tooth movement which may be undertaken.

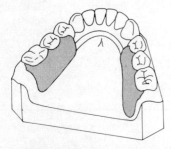

An alternative design of base plate incorporating a lingual bar.

and particularly in the area of the lingual fraenum, discomfort and ulceration will occur.

Undercut

There are usually undercuts on the lingual side of the lower alveolus, especially in the molar and premolar region. If the acrylic is extended into these areas during manufacture the appliance can only be removed from the work model by breaking the plaster and it can only be fitted after considerable trimming. Since the tags of molar clasps are embedded into this area they may become loose during such trimming. Undercuts should therefore be eliminated by waxing or plastering before the appliance is constructed. Alternatively the wire tags can be shaped so that they are largely out of the undercut area which may then be trimmed away in the laboratory at the end of construction.

Physical Limitations

The form and situation of the lower alveolus dictate that the acrylic base plate will consist of a 'U' shaped strip of plastic which runs parallel to the roots of the teeth. This is obviously very different from the situation in the upper arch and if the acrylic has to be trimmed to allow movement of a tooth it is very easy to weaken the appliance so that fracture occurs readily. In situations like this the appliance must be thickened in places during construction to allow for subsequent necessary trimming.

Acrylic form.

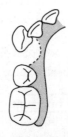 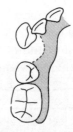

Incorrect, the necessary trimming to allow retraction of the canine will weaken the appliance.

Correct, the appliance has been thickened during construction so that trimming can be carried out.

If during the retraction of teeth any anchorage slip occurs, slight labial movement of the appliance may take place causing trauma to the gingivae lingual to the lower incisors and to the mucosa overlying the alveolus in this area. For this reason some operators prefer to replace the anterior part of the base plate with a lingual bar. This, however, has the disadvantage of reducing the number of teeth and area of mucosa available for anchorage support.

Retention

Lower appliances have poorer retention than uppers. This is partly because of the lack of palatal support but also because the shape of many of the lower teeth is usually less favourable for clasping.

The buccal aspect of the lower first molar presents a sloping rectangular surface and little undercut is obtainable. The conventional Adams' clasp is more difficult to fit and adjust satisfactorily than in the upper arch. In this situation a mesial and distal arrowhead in 0.8 mm wire are often more satisfactory. A pair of these on a tooth resembles an Adams' clasp with the bridge removed and the arrowheads pinched closed. Without the bridge the arrowheads can be adjusted to engage the undercut at the mesial and distal surfaces and the added thickness of the wire compensates for the lack of bridge and provides the clasps with added rigidity. A pair of such arrowheads on each lower first molar gives a good basis for retention and an additional clasp further forwards, perhaps an Adams' clasp on a first premolar or canine, will resist any displacement produced by activation of the appliance. It also gives a purchase where a finger tip may be applied to assist in removal of the appliance. When a clasp cannot be applied in this position an Adams' clasp in 0.6 mm wire can be placed on a lower incisor and, if well constructed, will give good retention.

Design of Springs

Lingual springs. The shape of the lower base plate has already been mentioned. In order to accommodate a sufficient length of spring to give the required flexibility, a lingual spring must have its coil well down the lingual acrylic and the wire must rise vertically up to the height of the gingival margin before turning through a right angle to engage the tooth. During activation the height of the spring is difficult to control because it will vary as the tooth moves. (This can be compared to the behaviour of one half of a bucket handle when the handle is raised or lowered.) As the arm of the spring varies from the vertical there is progressively more change in

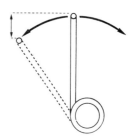

Activation of a lingual finger spring will cause the point of its application on the tooth to vary in height.

59

A suitable design of spring for the retraction of a mesially inclined and buccally placed canine.

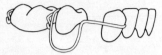

A plain loop emerging from the distal aspect of the second premolar.

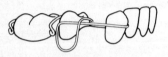

A reversed loop emerging from the mesial aspect of the second premolar.

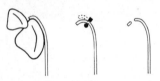

The simplest method for activating a buccal canine spring is to curve the end inwards and shorten the wire slightly.

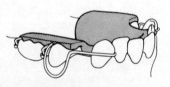

A suitable design of appliance to retract mesially placed canines.
Buccal springs in 0.7 mm wire are used and retention is provided by single arrowhead clasps in 0.8 mm wire on lower first molars. Shallow posterior bite planes are incorporated to gag the bite and facilitate correction of the canines.

height for a given amount of activation along the arch. Because of this it is sensible to use these springs only for comparatively small movements of teeth.

Buccal springs (0.7 mm wire). The sulcus surrounding the lower arch is shallow and designs of buccal springs, such as those commonly used in the upper, are less well tolerated. Springs such as those shown are well tolerated and useful in the retraction of canines. Activation is best carried out by curving the end of the spring inward and cutting off a short piece of wire. It is better not to adjust at the loop, as this moves the active end of the spring occlusally and secondary adjustment is required. The spring should be flexed lingually so that it engages on the canine and if the tooth is initially outstanding this assists in moving it into line.

If lingual or buccal movement is required springs similar to those described in the section on upper appliances (Chapter 4) may be used. Lower buccal springs should as a rule be kept shallower than in the upper arch. There may be some difficulty in accommodating lingual springs because a lingually positioned tooth may interfere with insertion of the appliance, particularly once the spring is activated.

Examples of Design

A Passive Appliance

A simple design with mesial and distal arrowheads in 0.8 mm wire on first molars will usually be adequate to act as a space maintainer. If poor retention is expected then a clasp placed further forwards will help to stabilize the appliance.

Sometimes teeth which might have improved their position naturally by drifting into adjacent spaces are prevented from doing so by the occlusion (e.g. a buccally placed lower canine trapped outside the upper arch). Occlusal interference may also hinder active fixed appliance movement of an upper tooth across the bite. In either case the use of a passive lower appliance carrying shallow posterior bite planes can relieve the occlusion and permit correction.

Active Appliances

A similar design to that described above can be used with the addition of buccal springs to retract canines. If a spring is only required on one side of the appliance then an additional clasp on the other side will help stability but where bilateral springs are required this will not be possible. An incisal clasp could be used in such a situation if necessary.

If slight distal movement of a first permanent molar is required, perhaps after the loss of a lower second molar to allow space for a premolar to erupt, then good clasping will be necessary. This manoeuvre could be carried out with a finger spring and clasping would then be to the first molar on the opposite side and bilaterally further forwards. The spring, in 0.6 mm wire can be brought up against the distal edge of the acrylic.

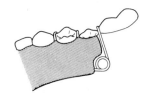

A suitable design of spring in 0.6 mm wire to carry out slight distal movement of a first molar providing space for a crowded second premolar.

An alternative way to carry out this movement would be by means of a screw and it would then be possible to clasp lower first molars and also to have bilateral clasps further forward. Activation of the screw would enlarge the premolar space. In either case care must be taken to minimize forward movement of anchor teeth. Activation of a spring should be kept at about one third of a premolar width and a screw should not be turned more than one quarter revolution per week. Anchorage loss is almost inevitable if a large amount of movement is attempted.

In rare situations an appliance can be used to align lower incisors. If no rotations or apical malpositions are present this will usually be unnecessary as spontaneous alignment may occur when space is made. The appliance would have a labial bow emerging from the distal aspects of the canines with medium sized loops. Stops can be placed mesial to the canines if they have previously been retracted. A fairly rigid spring in 0.7 mm wire can be placed lingual to the lower incisors and very gently advanced as the labial bow is activated, so that the lower incisors are squeezed into position. It should be stressed that such an appliance would not be used to alter the antero-posterior position of the lower incisors but merely to reduce imbrication.

THE LOWER REMOVABLE SECTIONAL APPLIANCE

Crowding and irregularity of the lower incisors present a special problem in orthodontics. A patient may attend with an otherwise good occlusion but with irregularity of the mandibular anterior teeth which is unacceptable. Such a patient may have had no previous orthodontic treatment or have had a course of treatment some years previously which may even have included extractions. This problem occurs commonly in young adults. Alignment of lower incisors is difficult with conventional removable appliances while fixed appliances may be unacceptable to such patients. In these circumstances the sectional removable appliance described by Barrer may be useful.*

Lower incisors have a mean collective mesio-distal width of 22 mm (± 1.4 mm). The enamel thickness of an incisor at the contact point is 0.75 mm. The removal of 50 per cent of the enamel from each contact point will create 3 mm of space in the incisor region. Such space may be used to effect incisor alignment if crowding is not too great and provided that any rotations are minimal.

*Barrer, H.G. (1975) *J.C.O.* 9, 486.

Enamel Stripping

This may be carried out before or after appliance construction, but is best done beforehand if the appliance can be supplied within a few days. Enamel removal may be carried out in several ways. Because the contact points will be tight initially it should be started with metal backed abrasive strips. When adequate access has been gained further enamel may be removed either in the same manner or with a mechanical aid if the operator prefers.

Safe sided discs, or specially designed reciprocating abraders are alternatives.

Appliance Construction

The lower incisor teeth are cut off the model. If contact point reduction has not been started clinically, then appropriate plaster must be removed from the teeth at this stage. A Vernier gauge will ensure that the correct amount of tooth reduction is carried out.

The teeth are set up to the anticipated new position and waxed in place. By using cold cure acrylic to construct the appliance the need to duplicate the wax up in plaster is avoided.

A 0.7 mm stainless steel wire is laid down. This should lie in close contact with the labial surfaces of the incisors, and pass around the gingival margin of the canine without contacting the gingivae or tooth. It should then pass over the canine-premolar contact point to again follow the gingival margin of the canine without contacting it. Finally the wire should finish lingually in the mid-line.

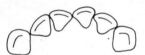

Incisal crowding before inter-proximal stripping.

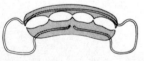

The sectional appliance, occlusal view.

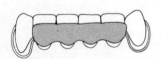

The sectional appliance in position.

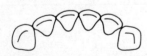

The corrected tooth position.

Cold cure acrylic 2 to 3 mm in thickness is laid down over the wire buccally and lingually. It extends no further than the distal surfaces of the laterals. Dentine coloured acrylic is aesthetically most acceptable.

Clinical Treatment

The appliance is inserted and adjusted to ensure suitable activation. Because the teeth have been moved in making the working model the appliance will probably not require activation at this stage. The patient is instructed to wear the appliance full-time except for meals.

At subsequent appointments activation can be carried out by adjusting the distal wire loops so as to approximate further the lingual and labial acrylic bars. Where local adjustments are necessary appropriate trimming and the addition of small areas of cold cure acrylic will be effective.

When tooth movement is complete the passive appliance will serve as a retainer. It may be worn full time at first and then only at nights. Finally it may be withdrawn altogether when stability seems assured. Long retention will be necessary if any rotations have been corrected.

CHAPTER 8

Fitting a Removable Appliance for the First Time

An appliance should ideally be fitted as soon as possible after the impression has been taken. Although a good fit is frequently achieved even after a delay of a month or more such a delay is inadvisable and must certainly be avoided if extractions have already been carried out. If there is any doubt about the patient's future co-operation it is good practice to fit the appliance and let it be worn for a visit or two prior to the extractions. The tasks to be carried out when the appliance is fitted may be grouped under two headings:

1. To prepare the appliance;
2. To instruct the patient.

PREPARATION

It should become second nature when picking up a new appliance for the first time to run the fingers over the base plate, and particularly over the fitting surface, checking for any sharp areas. Roughness of the acrylic may occur on the fitting surface as a result of air bubbles on the surface of the model. These areas can be quickly smoothed as can any sharp ends of wire. The appliance can then be checked quickly against the mouth and tried into position.

Fit of the Appliance

There are several possible reasons why an appliance may not fit.

The Wrong Appliance

This may seem a frivolous suggestion but in a busy practice or laboratory muddles can occur.

Anticipation of the Extractions

If the technician has removed from the model the teeth which are to be extracted and encroached on this area the appliance will not fit without modification until the extractions have been carried out. Acrylic can be readily trimmed away from the area which the tooth occupies but the correction of wirework encroaching on this area is more difficult. Except in cases where wires have to be positioned across extraction spaces the technician should be asked to leave all existing teeth on the model during appliance construction.

Eruption of Teeth

The eruption of palatally placed teeth, particularly upper second premolars, can cause problems. It is usually only troublesome if there has been some delay since the impression was taken. Unless the embedded parts of the wirework overlay the erupting teeth the acrylic can simply be trimmed away. Once again alteration of the wirework provides greater difficulty and the eruption of an instanding tooth should, in any case, have been foreseen during the planning of treatment.

Delay Since the Impression

Apart from allowing the eruption of further teeth delay in fitting an appliance allows forward movement of buccal teeth following orthodontic extractions or natural loss of deciduous molars and may interfere with fitting.

Subsequent Appliances

Occasionally a subsequent appliance will not fit because movement of the teeth has occurred since the impression was taken. This may result either because the previous appliance was left active or because the patient has thought that the appliance has completed its task and has ceased to wear it. Either of these events can cause great inconvenience and the latter can even produce the situation where neither the new nor the old appliance will fit.

Faulty Procedures

Faults can occur in the surgery or in the laboratory during construction of the appliance.

Impressions which are inadequately extended or those with air blows, drags, or which have been removed from the mouth before being fully set are obviously unlikely to give the best results. Neither will adequate impressions which have subsequently come away from the tray or been allowed to dry out. Over trimming of the models during the construction of Adams' clasps can make these clasps too tight so that insertion is impossible. Wire loops which lies close to the gingivae may not take account of the path of insertion so that they impinge on areas such as the canine eminence, particularly when this is bulbous, and prevent fitting.

Retention

This should always be checked carefully. If the appliance is well made little adjustment will be necessary. It should snap easily into place with gentle finger pressure and be a firm fit although readily removable. Retention may be poor because the appliance is badly designed to resist the displacing forces to which it is subjected. Attention to design should avoid this.

Adjustment of Clasps

Clasps made according to Adams' design offer good retention. Frequently, however, the operator is presented with an appliance on which the clasps are faulty and adjustment will be necessary.

When adjusting clasps the operator should avoid, as far as possible, bending the wire at the points where it has already been bent by the technician during construction. The only exception to this rule is that where the clasps are initially obviously too tight to permit insertion it may be necessary to grip each arrowhead in turn with the pliers and bend it outwards. Once the appliance can be seated (if necessary with the support of a finger) the accurate positioning of the arrowheads can be investigated. Possible faults are as follows:

Horizontal. The arrowheads do not contact the tooth or else grip it too tightly.

Vertical. The arrowheads grip too far occlusally or else push into the gingivae.

These faults can be corrected in most cases by a combination of bends at two points. Bending the wire just beyond the point where it has passed over the embrasure controls the height of the arrowhead. Bending the wire just

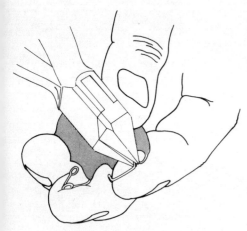

It is possible to adjust the clasp by flexing the arrowhead itself. Although this is generally not recommended it may allow a clasp with badly placed arrowheads to be salvaged.

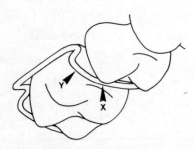

Ill fitting clasps can frequently be remedied by bending the wire at two points. Adjustment at *X* moves the arrowhead vertically. Adjustment at *Y* moves it horizontally.

short of the arrowhead controls its bucco-lingual position.

Take as an example a clasp which is found to have its arrowhead pushing into the gingivae. The wire can be bent at point X to move the arrowhead occlusally. The height can be corrected but the adjustment will also have the effect of moving the arrowhead away from the tooth. A bend can then be placed at point Y to compensate for this.

Correction of the Adams' clasp.

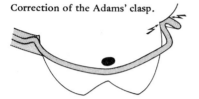
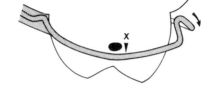
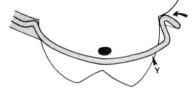

The arrowhead is pushing into the gingivae.

The first adjustment relieves the trauma but also moves the wire away from the tooth.

The second adjustment restores tooth contact but with the arrowhead at the correct height.

If the arrowhead grips the tooth too far occlusally it can be moved bucally by an adjustment at point Y. A further adjustment at point X will then bring it into contact at the correct position.

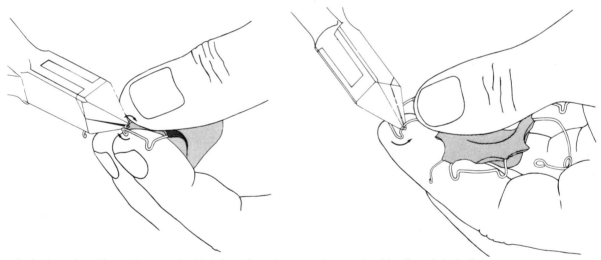

The horizontal position of the arrowhead is being adjusted to clear the tooth. Pressure from the finger and thumb limits vertical change.

The arrowhead is adjusted gingivally into the correct position for the sake of clarity the manoeuvre is shown on the opposite clasp.

It is important that the clasp does not grip the tooth tightly and an undercut of 0.25 mm has been shown to give an adequate clasp. It is useless to attempt to tighten the clasp by bending the wire at the point where it emerges from the plastic. This will merely interfere with the passage of the

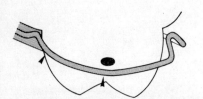

Adjustment between these two points is not recommended except where the clasp has to be recontoured over the contact point.

wire across the embrasure and prevent full seating of the appliance. The only indication for adjustment at this point occurs in a case where the wire passes high over the embrasure and interferes with the occlusion.

Many inadequate clasps can be corrected by the procedure described above but if the clasp is really hopeless then it may be necessary to replace it or have the appliance reconstructed.

Poor retention may be due to a conically shaped tooth and this is especially common when second molars are being clasped. Such potential difficulty should be noticed at the design stage and if possible an alternative design of appliance used.

Adjustments of Active Wirework

The appliance should now be easy to fit and have adequate retention. Labial wires, loops and springs can now be adjusted so that they are at the correct height and do not traumatize the cheeks, lips or gingivae.

Adjustments to the Acrylic

Apart from initial trimming to permit insertion some adjustments to the base plate may be necessary.

The acrylic will need to be trimmed to permit active tooth movement. This is of great importance and is frequently overlooked. The appliance should be inspected *in situ* to ensure that no part of the acrylic contacts the tooth to be moved and that the anticipated tooth movement will not re-establish this contact before the next visit. It is also very sensible to trim to allow desirable passive movement, e.g. to permit an outstanding canine to drop into line.

Bite Planes

Any excessive thickness may need to be reduced and a bite plane adjusted to give even contacts. In the case of posterior bite planes careful trimming will usually be necessary to ensure that the bite is evenly distributed. An anterior bite plane will need to be undermined before overjet reduction.

Appliance Activation

During the first few days with a new appliance the patient has to get used to inserting it correctly and must adapt to its presence and put up with a mild degree of discomfort. It is a sensible idea either to insert the appliance so that it is passive or to provide only slight activation so that it is self-activating and the springs cannot readily slip into the wrong position. If extra oral support is contemplated the appliance should certainly be fitted passively and the headgear added at the next visit.

INSTRUCTING THE PATIENT

When initial adjustments have been carried out the patient should be shown the appliance out of the mouth and *in situ*. The position of springs etc. can be pointed out and the correct method of insertion and removal should be taught.

Insertion

The appliance should be placed into the mouth and the anterior part put lightly into position with any springs in the correct place. If there is an anterior clasp or fitted wire it helps to locate the appliance. Firm upward pressure is then applied to the centre of the acrylic palate with fingers or thumb and the appliance should seat into position. It may finally be necessary to position buccally placed wires, such as buccal canine retractors or clips engaging buccal tubes, with the fingers. On no account should the appliance be bitten into position.

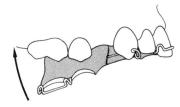

The correct method of insertion is to engage the anterior wire on the incisors and then press the acrylic palate upwards until the molar clasps engage. Removal is accomplished by pulling down on the molar clasps before disengaging the anterior teeth.

Removal

This is carried out in the reverse order. The fingertips are used to pull down on the bridges of the molar clasps until they disengage from the teeth. The front part of the appliance should then disengage readily. It is important that the posterior part is not pulled down excessively or the anterior wire may be flexed and distorted. Similarly if the clasp on one side of the appliance is pulled well down before the other, then distortion of the clasp which is still engaged may occur.

The patient should be given an opportunity to practise removal and insertion of the appliance under supervision until it is certain that this can be carried out satisfactorily.

Information

There are arguments for and against the use of printed hand-outs. The spoken word may be quickly forgotten: elaborate printed instructions may not be read. The best compromise is probably to give simple verbal instructions backed up with more printed information. The patient should be instructed to wear the appliance full-time, i.e. all day, all night, for meals and as far as possible for sports. Wear during meals is most important, particularly if bite opening has to be achieved or if teeth are being moved across the bite. As far as possible cleaning should be carried out after meals and particular care should be given to cleaning the fitting surface of the appliance, either with a nail brush or with the patient's own tooth brush. If, on occasion, circumstances do not permit this then the appliance should at least be removed from the mouth and rinsed under a tap. If it does prove necessary to remove the appliance other than for cleaning, e.g. during vigorous sports or the playing of a wind instrument the patient should be instructed to place it in a rigid container such as a tobacco tin, which will protect it from accidental damage.

The patient will be very aware initially of the large bulk of the appliance and will probably experience excess salivation and difficulty in swallowing. Reassurance should be given that this is quite normal and that the appliance will rapidly feel more comfortable. Difficulties with excessive salivation and swallowing usually disappear within a few hours. Normal speech may take 24 to 48 hours to achieve. The most difficult adaptation is to accept the wear of the appliance at meal times and this may well take several days to accomplish. The patient should be encouraged to persevere until this has been achieved.

It is not necessary to give the patient complex instructions about diet. A normal diet can usually be enjoyed during the period of treatment. It is only necessary to avoid certain sticky confections such as toffees and chewing gum.

Finally, it is important that in the event of pain, trauma to the soft tissue, breakage, etc., the patient should contact the practice at once and be seen as soon as possible so that wear is not interrupted. If the appliance can be tolerated for at least part of the time it will help to maintain the fit until it can be adjusted. It is a good idea to give a small amount of soft red carding wax to the patient when the appliance is fitted. A small piece stuck over a wire loop which is causing irritation during the first few days will often allow the patient to adapt and save an extra visit to the surgery. Alternatively it may permit an otherwise unwearable appliance to be tolerated until the patient can return.

CHAPTER 9

Management of Treatment Progress

Throughout the course of active treatment the patient will usually attend monthly. There are exceptions to this. We have said already that the interval between impression taking and fitting the appliance should be kept as short as possible. Similarly if an appliance is fitted passive it is frequently possible to carry out the first adjustment after as little as a week or two.

Longer intervals are adequate for passive appliances: space maintainers and retainers may be left unattended for several months if the patient is sensible and co-operative. It need hardly be said that breakages and other emergencies which prevent wear of the appliance must be dealt with without delay.

Despite these exceptions we can restate the general rule that a patient wearing an active appliance should be seen at approximately monthly intervals. More frequent visits are unproductive, longer intervals allow things to go wrong and prolong treatment. The patient's social and educational requirements may make regular orthodontic attendance difficult and compromises must sometimes be made. From time to time parents may make requests which are clinically unrealistic, e.g. that a child at boarding school should be seen only during vacations and occasionally at half-term. Such arrangements must be gently but firmly rejected.

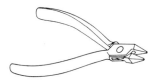

Adams' universal pliers.

EQUIPMENT

Relatively little equipment is required for the adjustment of removable appliances:

Adams' universal pliers;	(fig. IX 1)
spring-forming pliers;	(fig. IX 2)

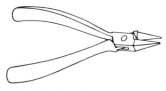

Spring-forming pliers.

wire cutters; (fig. IX 3)
dividers; (fig. IX 4)
engineer's Vernier gauge (alternative—a metal ruler);
grease pencil (Chinagraph type).

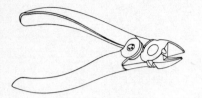

A stout pair of wire cutters is an essential aid.

Pliers

The two pairs of pliers listed will be found invaluable. They are robust and with a little care will give long service. We recommend the variety of pliers which have their working tips impregnated with tungsten carbide. The plier tips should always be reserved for adjusting lighter wires and if heavier wires, such as extra oral face bows, require adjustment, then an area of the beak nearer to the hinge should be used whenever possible. Some operators find a pair of concave/convex beaked pliers useful.

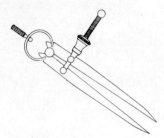

A pair of engineering spring dividers is another useful accessory.

We would recommend anyone with an urge to spend more money on pliers to buy an extra pair of the basic pliers, which we have described, rather than a pair designed for some specialised purpose. Most orthodontists seem to possess a collection of redundant pliers whose purchase 'seemed a good idea at the time'.

Maun Cutting Pliers

These are a robust pair of cutters whose design allows them to deal with orthodontic wires up to and including those used with extra oral traction.

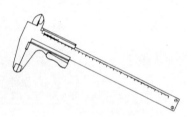

An engineer's Vernier gauge is extremely useful but a millimetre rule makes a cheaper alternative.

Measuring Instruments

A pair of engineering spring dividers (100—150 mm preferably stainless) is most useful, as is an engineer's Vernier gauge. A cheap alternative to the latter is a small metal ruler but it is important to make sure that the zero mark coincides with the end of the ruler, to facilitate the measurement of overjets.

A grease pencil of the Chinagraph type is a cheap and invaluable aid.

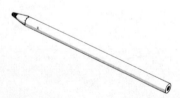

A grease pencil simplifies acrylic trimming and wire adjustment.

TASKS AT EACH VISIT

1. Assessment of Progress

A yachtsman setting out to sea can often check his position during the early stages of his voyage by referring back to the port which he is leaving. Once he is out of sight of land he

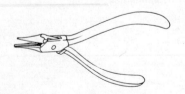

A pair of concave/convex beaked pliers may be found useful.

may look for fixed points against which he may judge his progress and he may also work out a 'dead reckoning' by keeping track of his direction and speed during each part of his voyage. As his eventual destination comes into sight he looks ahead for landmarks which will bring him safely into port.

During orthodontic treatment similar assessments may be made.

Retrospective Assessment

Progress may be assessed at any stage by reference to the starting position. It is obvious, therefore, that good records of this position are necessary.

Models. A pair of well trimmed correctly articulated models taken just before treatment commences is most important.

X-rays. Removable appliances do not allow apical control and if a case is correctly selected for treatment entirely with such appliances it is not usually necessary to have lateral skull cephalostat X-rays. This is fortunate, as many operators who carry out such simple treatment have no access to a cephalostat. It is, of course, assumed that adequate radiographic investigations of the patient will have been made at the time of diagnosis and if only part of the treatment is to be carried out with a simple removable appliance the rest of the treatment may still require that cephalostat X-rays are obtained.

Photographs. Photographic records are generally underutilized but can be a very valuable form of record. 35mm colour transparencies are easy to store and cheap by comparison with a set of study models.

These initial records are of use in assessing progress over the first few visits. Beyond this they provide a guide to general progress but as the occlusion alters with treatment they rapidly become of little use in assessing monthly improvement.

Current Assessment

The position of the teeth which are being moved should be recorded at each visit. A simple measurement is often sufficient e.g. during retraction of upper canines a pair of dividers

73

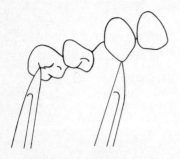

A suitable measurement to assess canine retraction. This would need to be considered together with a record of the overjet to make sure that anchorage loss was not occurring.

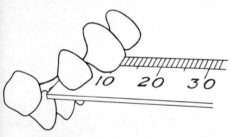

The method of overjet measurement using a millimetre rule.

may be used to measure the distance from the highest part of the buccal fissure of the first molar to the tip of the canine. The points of the dividers can then be pressed into the record card and the indentations labelled thus:

A record of the overjet should confirm that the upper incisors are not being pushed forwards by the acrylic base plate as a result of anchorage slip.

The operator should get into the habit of using the same points of reference as a routine, e.g. overjet measurements might be taken from the mesial tip of the upper left central incisor and when this routine must be changed, perhaps because the tooth in question is fractured or lost, then the position from which measurements have been taken should be noted carefully on the card. Particular difficulties may be experienced when a point of reference moves. This commonly occurs when extractions have been carried out in the lower arch and when, for example, a prominent lower incisor from which the overjet has been measured drops lingually as spontaneous incisor alignment occurs and creates an apparent increase in recorded overjet. Measurement is carried out using a ruler with a mm scale, with the zero point at the extreme end. It should be pointed out that overjet measurement is an arbitrary, rather than a defined, parameter and represents the horizontal distance between the labial surface of the lower incisors and the incisal edge of the uppers. Some variation is bound to occur as a result of different inclinations of the ruler but in practice this is small and the overjet measurement is reproducible.

Other factors may influence the overjet measurement. Extra oral traction to the upper jaw may cause a reduction in the overjet. The use of an anterior bite plane designed to permit molar eruption may rotate the mandible downwards and produce an increase in overjet.

Apparent changes in the overjet may be brought about by changes in mandibular posture associated with the wearing of the appliance.

A comparison of the molar occlusion with that of the original study models is also a useful guide to progress and changes can be noted on the record card. Here again, the operator may be deceived. Anchorage slip in the upper arch, which would normally cause an alteration of the molar occlusion, may be masked by slight mesial drift of the lower molar when lower premolar extractions have been carried out. Measurements such as those shown would help to keep track of such progressive changes in the lower arch:

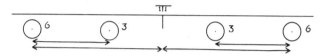

Considerable improvisation is possible in taking measurements. The vertical position of an erupting tooth may be recorded by measuring its height from a matchstick placed across the two neighbouring teeth. The width of extraction spaces may also be recorded using the Vernier gauge. Intercanine or interpremolar widths, for example, may be recorded to check on desired or unwanted bucco-lingual movement.

The object is to comprehend what movements are occurring and to provide a record against which the patient may be checked at a subsequent visit. Only by recording such changes will lack of progress or unwanted movement be detected and corrected at the earliest opportunity.

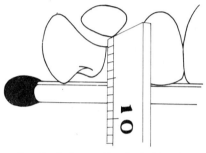

A method of measuring the height of a partially erupted canine.

Forward Projection

Towards the end of a particular tooth movement the operator will be able to judge progress by comparing the existing position with the desired final position.

Two obvious examples are: (1) during the final stages of canine retraction the question arises 'is there still enough space to obtain a Class I relationship with the lower arch?' and (2) during overjet reduction 'how does the amount of space available relate to the amount of space which will be required?'

2. Adjustment

Normal wear will usually cause some loosening of the appliance in the mouth between visits and alteration in the position of some of the wirework. Clasps may need to be tightened (see Chapter 8). Palatal finger springs which originally passed over the contact point may need to be

Spring adaptation.

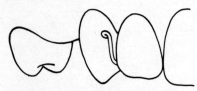

When the appliance is first fitted the spring may have to pass over the contact point between two teeth.

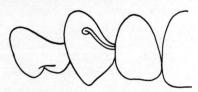

Once tooth movement has commenced the wire should be recontoured closer to the gingival margin.

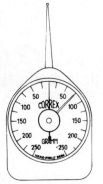

The 'Correx' force gauge.

contoured gingivally as soon as space permits. Repairs may be necessary and also adjustments to the base plate, such as trimming, or the addition of extra acrylic.

3. Activation

It is generally held that for a single rooted tooth a force of 30 to 50 g is appropriate to produce controlled movement with minimal tipping. The thickness and length of the spring will determine the amount of activation necessary to produce such a force, but a desirable activation is roughly one third to one half of a unit. A palatal finger spring constructed of 0.5 mm wire correctly activated will deliver the desired force.

If more activation is attempted the appliance may be difficult to insert correctly. The chance of the spring being wrongly positioned is increased and the spring is also more prone to damage.

A thicker or shorter spring may easily produce a force which is too heavy. For example, if a buccal canine retractor is constructed in 0.7 mm wire activation of less than a third of a unit is all that is permissible if the force is to be kept below 50 g. The tooth will quickly move through this distance and halt. Unless the patient attends frequently this produces slow movement and provides a temptation to over-activate the appliance. This may result in pain, anchorage slip and perhaps unwanted tilting of the tooth.

In general, palatal finger springs made in 0.5 mm wire to the design described are ideal and we favour the use of these wherever possible.

If the operator has access to a force gauge of the 'Correx' type it is possible to check the spring pressure being applied. This may be carried out in the following manner:

Palatal Springs

The appliance is placed in the mouth with the spring in the correct position. The point at the edge of the acrylic from which the spring emerges, is marked with a grease pencil. The point on the spring which delivers force to the tooth can also be marked.

The appliance is withdrawn from the mouth and activated. The arm of the force gauge can then be pushed against the spring to return it to the mark on the base plate. The force which will be delivered to the tooth can then be read.

76

Buccal Springs

A buccal spring can be checked by measuring the position of the spring tip relative to the mesial arrowhead of the molar clasp on that side. This can be done with a pair of spring dividers when the appliance is in the mouth. The appliance is removed from the mouth, and the arm of the force gauge again used to flex the spring back into its original place.

It is not necessary to measure force routinely in this manner, but it does help the operator to assess the sort of activation which will deliver the required force. Once this activation has been assessed it is still often useful to mark the position of a palatal finger spring with a grease pencil when the appliance is in position, or to measure the position of a buccal spring in the way described so that the actual amount of activation can be seen more easily.

Canine Retraction Springs

Activation is carried out by grasping the spring at the desired place with the plier beaks and flexing it with a finger or thumb until the required position is reached. During activation the spring is permanently deformed by bending it beyond its elastic limit.

It is good practice to avoid bending the spring at places where the wire has been bent during its formation and also to avoid carrying out successive activations at the same position. Apart from trying to avoid breakages it should be remembered that activation of a spring offers a chance to modify the direction of tooth movement.

An appliance may sometimes be constructed with the coils of canine finger springs, for example, placed too far distally. Simple activation of the spring from the coil will

Remember that a spring need not always be activated at the same point.

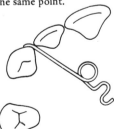

The initial position of a palatal finger spring.

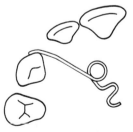

The spring has been cranked along its length to limit buccal movement of the canine.

The assessment of spring activation.

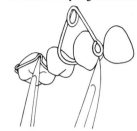

The dividers are used in the mouth to measure the distance of the point of application of a buccal spring from a convenient land mark such as the mesial arrowhead of the molar clasp.

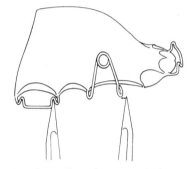

When the appliance is compared with the same measurement out of the mouth the degree of spring activation can be seen.

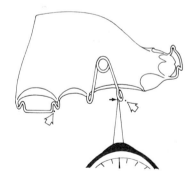

The force may be assessed by using the gauge to flex the spring back to its active position. This may be judged against divider marks indicated on a piece of paper.

77

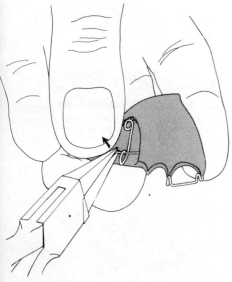

A buccal canine spring being flexed with the finger to provide activation.

Adjustment to the guard may be necessary to permit free movement of the spring.

move the canine buccally as it is retracted. A crank progressively placed into the spring will provide activation and help to limit this tendency. When such cranking is not necessary the bend should be placed near to the coil of the spring.

In the case of a buccal spring it will often be necessary to adjust the spring at more than one point. The wire can be bent near to where it emerges on the buccal side of the arch so that the coil is correctly positioned. The coil itself can then be grasped in the beaks of the spring-forming pliers and the free end flexed with the thumb to the desired position.

Secondary Adjustments

In either case, further adjustments may be necessary. In the case of a palatal finger spring, the height may need adjustment so that the spring rests just clear of the gingival margin. If the wire projects too far buccally it may cause trauma to the cheek and require shortening. If a guard is being used care must be taken to see that the spring slides freely.

A buccal spring may also require adjustment for height and it may be necessary to flex the free end of the spring inwards with the thumb so that it engages the tooth firmly, or sometimes to flex the entire spring inwards if the coil is too prominent.

When such adjustments have had to be carried out it is necessary to re-check that the spring activation has not been inadvertently altered.

Labial Wires

The general principle of avoiding existing bends during activation and of carrying out the adjustment at different points still applies. Where the incisors are irregular it may be necessary to combine activation of the labial wire with careful selective trimming of the palatal acrylic. The wire may also be kinked to bring pressure to bear on a particular tooth and so help in obtaining alignment.

Again, it is possible to measure activation of anterior wires and this can be done by drilling a small pin-hole into the acrylic of the anterior bite plane and measuring from this to the mid-line point on the labial wire which can be marked with a grease pencil. The difference between this measurement with the appliance in and out of the mouth will show the amount of activation. A spring gauge can be used to measure the force being delivered.

The labial bow. This is activated by reducing the size of the loops. Each side is dealt with individually by holding the loop in the pliers and flexing the bow mesial to them. Some operators find that a pair of concave/convex beaked pliers is useful for this. With either method it will be necessary to

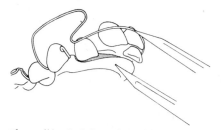

If a small bur hole is made in the anterior bite plane it may be used to locate one point of a pair of dividers and allow the activation of a labial wire to be assessed.

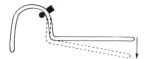

Closure of the adjustment loop moves the labial bow occlusally. Secondary adjustment will be necessary.

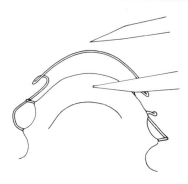

readjust the vertical height of the labial wire because closure of the loops will cause this to move occlusally. If the incisors are notably proclined this occlusal activation may be desirable as it will help to combat the tendency of the activated labial bow to slide up towards the gingivae. It may also be necessary to flex the loops inwards or outwards as required to avoid trauma to the lip or alveolus respectively.

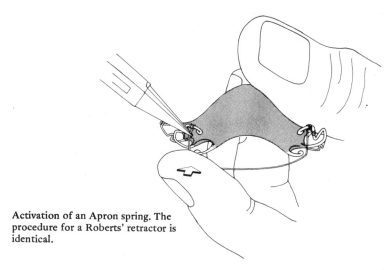

Activation of an Apron spring. The procedure for a Roberts' retractor is identical.

Light wires. Light wires such as the Apron spring and Roberts' retractor again need activation on each side. The wire should be gripped near to the top of the descending vertical arm and the spring flexed palatally. Vertical adjustment is usually unnecessary but the supporting arms may again need bucco-palatal adjustment so that trauma is avoided.

Springs Carrying Out Lingual Movements

Buccal springs (described in Chapter 4) to move teeth palatally can be adjusted in a similar manner to that described for buccal canine springs. A buccal canine spring can itself be used to push the tooth palatally, perhaps at the end of retraction. To achieve this the foot of the spring which engages the tooth is bent through 90° and the spring adapted so that this can rest on the buccal face of the canine.

Springs Carrying Out Buccal Movement

Cranked palatal finger springs can be adjusted in the manner described for palatal finger springs. 'T' springs are useful for pushing premolars buccally and can be activated simply by seizing the crosspiece of the 'T' and pulling the spring outwards and slightly away from the fitting surface of the acrylic so that it binds on the tooth during insertion. The provision of extra loops allows for further adjustment of the spring as the tooth moves.

'Z' springs are useful for proclining individual incisors. Again the wire is gripped in the pliers and pulled forwards and slightly upwards from the acrylic to activate it. By flexing the spring in this manner the appliance is self-activating as it is put into the mouth and any tendency for the spring to be trapped over the incisal edge of the tooth by the acrylic is avoided.

Acrylic

Adjustments to acrylic may be required from time to time. At each visit it is important to check that the teeth being moved are free from contact with the base plate and likely to remain so at least until the next appointment. When carrying out any trimming to accomplish this it must be remembered that allowance has to be made for the soft tissue which may be heaped up in advance of a moving tooth.

Anterior planes may need to be built up to continue bite-opening or possibly to make-good occlusal wear. During incisor retraction acrylic will need to be trimmed from the fitting surface to permit tooth movement.

Posterior planes may need to be repaired during use as small fragments break away. They are trimmed to reduce the degree of bite opening as successful tooth movement

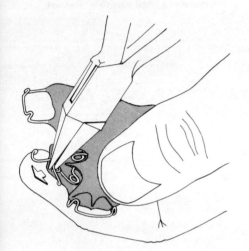

Activation of a 'Z' spring . The spring is pulled upward and labially so that both coils are activated.

occurs. Such reduction is usually carried out during two successive visits and preceeds the total removal of the occlusal cover.

Occasionally it may be possible to remove occlusal cover entirely at one appointment when a tooth in crossbite has corrected sufficiently to allow the posterior teeth into occlusion without trauma to the newly moved tooth.

4. General Dental Care

The state of the oral hygiene must be borne in mind at each appointment and any deficiencies pointed out to the patient and corrected. It is also wise from time to time to check that the patient's visits to the general practitioner for routine inspections and treatment are being continued.

CHAPTER 10

Extra Oral Forces

Most multiband appliance systems make extensive use of extra oral forces. By comparison such forces are much less used with removable appliances. There is no good clinical reason why this should be so. Extra oral forces can readily be adapted for use in removable appliance orthodontics and can extend considerably the range of treatment which can be undertaken.

TRACTION OR ANCHORAGE

An operator who is employing extra oral forces may try to distinguish between extra oral traction and extra oral anchorage. The former expression implies that teeth are being moved distally to gain space, e.g. distal movement of upper molars to accommodate mildly crowded canines in an occlusion which is otherwise normal. The latter expression merely suggests that the force is stabilizing teeth which are themselves being used for anchorage, e.g. the prevention of mesial movement of upper molars during canine retraction.

The essential difference between these functions is quantitative rather than qualitative. Clinically they are difficult to differentiate. In the example just given it is possible to apply headgear to move upper molar teeth distally and then continue its application while canines and premolar teeth are retracted. In theory this makes a change from traction to anchorage, yet the headgear remains unchanged. It may be that a patient who still wears headgear with enthusiasm during the second phase of treatment will continue to move the molars distally.

ORTHOPAEDIC EFFECTS

It is possible that heavy extra oral force applied for a substantial proportion of each day to a patient who is growing

82

rapidly may have an 'orthopaedic' effect. In addition to distal movement of teeth through bone there could be a restraint on maxillary growth. This would be favourable in a Class II case with an underlying skeletal discrepancy.

HEADGEAR ATTACHMENT

Headgear can be applied either directly to a removable appliance or indirectly to molar bands over which the appliance is clipped.

Direct Attachment to the Appliance

Many different patterns of headgear are available ranging from full headcap with anterior high pull traction to a neck strap delivering cervical traction. When headgear is applied directly to a removable appliance the direction of pull should be parallel to the occlusal plane or from above it. A force from below the occlusal plane, such as is delivered from a neck strap, exerts a downward force on the appliance and tends to unseat it. For this reason we recommend the use of full headgear when applying force directly to a removable appliance.

The headgear force may be applied to the removable appliance in several ways:

The Integral Face Bow

The appliance may be constructed with a face bow as an integral part but unless the patient is prepared to accept full time headgear wear such an appliance is essentially a part time one. This method is, therefore, only of limited application.

'J' Hooks

It is possible to apply a high-pull headgear force to the front of a removable appliance in a similar manner to that in which it is sometimes used with fixed appliances. Such an arrangement is useful in deep overbite cases or where retention is poor, e.g. in first molar extraction cases, because the upward pull makes a contribution to the retention of the appliance. This type of headgear can be obtained complete with 'J' hooks. A suitable rigid labial wire must be incorporated into the appliance and this should have loops or soldered hooks for the engagement of the 'J' hooks. A disadvantage of this method is that in cases in which an overjet has to be reduced

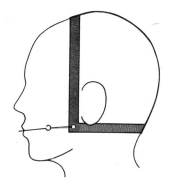

A full headcap delivering the force parallel to the occlusal plane.

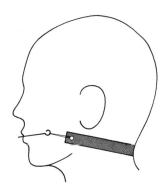

A neck strap delivering the force from below the occlusal plane. Although suitable for attachment via molar bands it will tend to produce displacement if attached directly to a removable appliance.

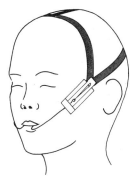

A high-pull headcap can be attached to the front of an appliance.

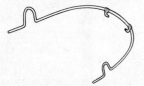

It is necessary to make special provision for the attachment of 'J' hooks during overjet reduction.

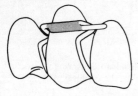

following canine retraction a flexible labial bow is insufficiently rigid to accept a high pull force. An alternative method of application is necessary during overjet reduction. This could be provided by using a detachable, stopped buccal arch, which engages into tubes soldered to the Adams' clasps and carries loops anteriorly for the 'J' hooks. An alternative method is to replace the stops of canines with Adams' clasps. These can carry soldered spurs which project forward to provide an attachment for the 'J' hooks.

Hooks soldered to a labial wire permit the engagement of 'J' hooks.

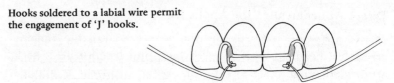

Soldered Tubes to Adams' Clasps

This is probably the best known method of attachment of extra oral force to removable appliances. It can be used with Adams' clasps on premolars and second molars as well as its more usual use on first molars. Attachment to the first molars is most satisfactory in practice. A length of stainless steel tube is soldered to the bridge of the Adams' clasp. To avoid trauma and discomfort this tube should be sited above the bridge rather than buccally, and for the same reason its ends must be chamfered and smoothed. The internal diameter will be determined by the gauge of the face bow (commonly 1.15 mm).

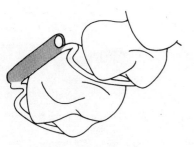

An Adams' clasp carrying a soldered tube for the attachment of a face bow.

Indirect Attachment of Headgear via Molar Bands

An alternative method of combining extra oral techniques with removable appliance therapy is to use tubes welded onto molar bands. The removable appliance is then retained in place by means of clips which engage over these tubes. A small stock of preformed molar bands will provide bands of the correct size for most patients. These bands may be purchased with suitable round tubes welded by the supplier. Alternatively plain bands may be used and the tubes welded by the technician in the laboratory. The bands, complete with their tubes, are cemented to the anchor molars and the impression for the work model taken over them. The technician can then construct a suitable removable appliance to be fitted at the next appointment.

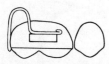

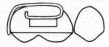

Two methods of providing retention of a removable appliance when the molars are banded, 0.7 mm wire is used.

84

This technique has a number of advantages:

1. Distal movement of the molars may be carried out using only the headgear and molar bands prior to fitting the first removable appliance.

2. If the first molars have been lost, bands provide a more secure retention to the second molars than the conventional Adams' clasps.

3. Should the operator so wish, it is possible to use a simple cervical strap without risk of displacing the appliance.

4. Molar rotation can be corrected initially.

5. It may be desired to finish a case with a fixed appliance following the retraction of buccal teeth with a removable appliance. In such a case double buccal tubes can be used on the molar bands and the same headgear continued through both phases of treatment.

THE FACE BOW

The face bow consists of an inner arch which engages the molar tubes and which is soldered in the midline to a heavier outer arch or whisker. The ends of the whisker are bent into hooks to take the extra oral force. Face bows may be constructed by the technician for each case or obtained preformed by the manufacturer in a number of sizes and wire gauges. We prefer preformed bows as they are less likely to fracture during use and should breakage occur they can be quickly replaced from stock. Furthermore, they can be sterilized at the end of treatment and reused for other cases.

The inner bow is available in several wire diameters. It is essential to avoid confusion by standardizing on a single diameter. We suggest 1.15 mm is adequate for all cases. Stops must be provided to deliver the force to the molar tubes and hold the front of the bow away from the incisors. Welded stops or bayonet bends may achieve this but vertical loops are suitable and have the added advantage of allowing easy adjustment of the inner bow as treatment progresses. Preformed bows can be obtained with the inner arch in four or five sizes, so that if a small stock is maintained most arch lengths can be quickly accommodated. The outer bow is manufactured in two or three lengths. We would suggest standardizing on a short or medium size and it is useful to order bows with ready bent hooks.

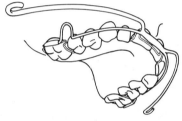

A typical face bow showing the method of attachment via molar tubes.

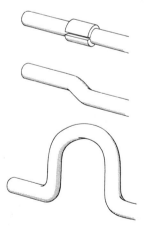

A stop must be provided where the inner arch enters the tube. This may take the form of a welded stop, a bayonet bend or a vertical loop.

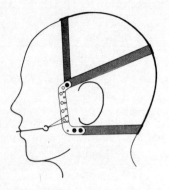

A typical adjustable headcap which may be quickly adapted to suit all sizes. It also allows the direction of the force to be varied.

THE HEADCAP

The headcap, like the face bow, may be made in the practice. Suitable materials for this are plastic tape or webbing, but alternatively headcaps may be bought preformed in a variety of patterns. Some are supplied in a range of sizes; others are adjustable. We would recommend the adjustable type to minimize the stock which must be kept.

ELASTIC FORCE

Although some headcaps deliver their force by means of specialized assemblies incorporating springs, we recommend the use of simple elastic traction. Standard stationery elastics are used and can be bought cheaply in bulk. It is not necessary to keep more than three or four sizes in stock. A selection from sizes 6 to 12 will be adequate for most purposes.

FITTING THE HEADGEAR

When the headgear is to be attached direct to the removable appliance by means of tubes on the molar clasps, it is good practice to fit the appliance first and add the extra oral components at the next visit. This allows the patient to adapt to the use of the removable appliance before learning to cope with the headgear.

Procedure

The correct size of face bow must first be selected. The work model will help in this selection and in any initial adaptation to the arch form. To complete the adaptation the bow should be fitted into one buccal tube and the relationship of the second side to its tube inspected. Adjustment of the first

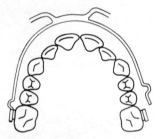

The face bow inserted on one side. Adjustment will be required as the other side is well clear of the tube.

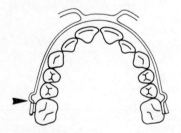

Adjustment at the point shown permits passive engagement in both tubes.

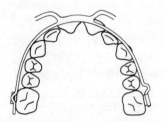

The face bow inserted on the second side. Without further adjustment the inner arch can still not be fitted passively.

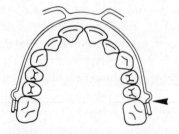

Adjustment at the point shown brings the second side level with its tube.

side is carried out until the second side is lying alongside, and level with, its tube. This process is then repeated with the bow inserted on the second side and usually produces an appliance which engages passively in both tubes, although some further minor adjustment may be required. It is important to check that the vertical loops do not impinge on the alveolus and, if necessary, they must be flared buccally. If the ends of the arch project through the molar tubes they may traumatize the buccal mucosa and must be shortened and smoothed. Finally it must be ensured that the junction of the inner and outer bow lies passively between the lips and that the outer bow lies parallel to the cheek.

A headcap should either be constructed or selected from stock and adjusted to a comfortable fit. The hooks for the elastics should lie just in front of the ears. A suitable size of elastic is chosen and fitted from the hook on the headcap to that on the face bow. The patient should be given a supply of these elastics because they will need to be changed every few days as their strength decreases.

HEADGEAR FORCES

There is no reliable rule of thumb to suggest the right force for the headgear. We suggest that an elastic which gives a force of about 500 g per side will be suitable to start with and as treatment proceeds this can be increased at the discretion of the patient by the use of more than one elastic. It is very unlikely that the patient will increase this to an unacceptable level as instability of the appliance or pain in the anchor teeth will discourage the use of excessive force.

A ready test of the stability of an appliance carrying a directly attached headgear can be made by asking the patient to open the mouth widely and tilt the head back to look at the ceiling. An appliance which remains secure during this manoeuvre is likely to be satisfactory. In a case where molar bands are used stability is not a problem.

HEADGEAR TIMING

Headgear success depends entirely on patient co-operation. It is therefore essential for the patient and parent to understand and accept the headgear as an important and integral part of treatment, and not as an optional extra. One should avoid giving the impression that the headgear is merely a bedtime appliance. It is better to introduce it to the patient pointing out that it need not be worn during school hours. The length of wear can easily be reduced later in treatment, but once a pattern of use has been established it may be difficult to extend the number of hours. For active distal movement a minimum of 12 hours a day will be necessary.

ASSESSMENT OF PROGRESS

At subsequent visits the success of the headgear must be assessed. If anchorage is slipping or desired distal movement is not occuring then the fault will lie either in the force level or in the hours of wear. (This assumes, of course, that the appliance is still a good fit in the mouth.) A headgear which has received regular wear will have lost its new appearance. Other clinical guides are variable and not always reliable, but points to watch for are:

1. The patient should be able to fit the headgear quickly without the use of a mirror.

2. The teeth to which the force is applied will show increased mobility and may be slightly sensitive to pressure, particularly in the early morning. (This applies especially where molar bands are being used.)

3. The patient's supply of elastics should be diminishing. One should be suspicious of the patient who rarely requires a further supply of elastics.

It is helpful to ask the patient to keep a chart of the hours of wear. Although this can readily be falsified it is often possible with practice to distinguish the genuine article from the forgery. Keeping such a chart in itself provides an incentive to the patient's enthusiasm and also makes it much easier for the operator to assess quickly the average length of wear which the headgear is receiving each day.

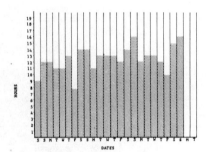

A typical headgear chart. A block diagram is easy for the patient to keep and provides an instant picture of co-operation.

CHAPTER 11

Fixed and Removable Appliances

Fixed appliances and removable appliances are fundamentally different and are appropriate to the solution of different problems. The use of both types may overlap, however, and they may be used in association to the advantage of some patients. Such combined use may arise in several ways:

1. A preliminary phase of treatment such as canine retraction may be carried out with a removable appliance and arch alignment completed with a fixed appliance.

2. A local irregularity such as the rotation of a single tooth may be corrected with a combination of fixed appliances and removable appliances.

3. A fixed appliance may be used in one arch while the other is treated by a removable appliance.

4. One technique of adding extra oral force to the removable appliance involves the use of at least molar bands.

UPPER REMOVABLE APPLIANCE AND LOWER FIXED APPLIANCE USED CONCURRENTLY

The scope of removable appliance therapy is undoubtedly much greater in the upper than in the lower arch. It is therefore often possible to apply upper removable appliances successfully while the problem in the lower arch requires a fixed appliance to achieve the necessary result. In using this combination the general principles of both will apply, but it is worth recalling that it is possible to use such additional techniques as headgear and Class II, or Class III elastic traction. In practice few operators would embark on such a treatment plan unless the treatment required in the upper was minimal, e.g. correction of an incisor crossbite or of a mesially tilted canine.

UPPER FIXED APPLIANCE AND LOWER REMOVABLE APPLIANCE USED CONCURRENTLY

For reasons outlined above, this combination is of very limited clinical value except in those cases where a lower bite raising appliance is of assistance to some upper arch tooth movement. There is no case for using a lower appliance with active components when an upper fixed appliance is in use.

UPPER FIXED APPLIANCE AND UPPER REMOVABLE APPLIANCE USED CONSECUTIVELY

This is a popular technique and is a two stage treatment which uses a removable appliance to carry out the distal movement of premolars and canines, followed by a fixed appliance to effect incisor alignment and space closure. Removable appliances provide an efficient method of moving buccal teeth distally without undue strain on the anchorage. This is particularly so when the teeth are mesially inclined at the commencement of treatment. The use of a fixed appliance during the final stage corrects the incisor malalignment. If premolars and canines are also banded then any necessary uprighting may be achieved during the finishing phase. If such a combination treatment plan is contemplated then it is probably wise to place first molar bands at the start of treatment and retain the removable appliance with clips over buccal tubes as described in Chapter 10.

UPPER FIXED APPLIANCE AND UPPER REMOVABLE APPLIANCE USED CONCURRENTLY

During the course of fixed appliance therapy it is sometimes helpful to prop open the bite. An example of this occurs when lingually occluding and palatally displaced upper canines are being corrected. A removable appliance carrying an anterior bite plane is constructed so as to clip over the molar tubes. As the canines move towards correct buccolingual relationship the bite plane may be progressively reduced in height before finally being discarded.

A similar removable bite plane may be helpful in the early stages of multiband therapy where there is a much increased overbite. Upper bands may be placed together with a bite plane to reduce the overbite. This permits the placement of lower incisor brackets without risk of trauma from the upper incisors.

The scope of removable appliance therapy may be considerably extended in some cases by the addition of a single band to a tooth. This is probably more true in recent years than formerly as the advent of direct bonding techniques allows the practitioner who does not wish to purchase a stock of bands to use these combinations. In this way a tooth may be extruded or rotated.

Extrusion

Correction of vertical displacements is not generally possible with removable appliances. Cases arise, however, where one or two teeth lie short of the occlusal level of the remaining teeth and must be moved into occlusion. This situation may occur in the case of a canine which has erupted ectopically. It may also arise following surgical exposure of a misplaced canine or a central incisor which has been displaced by a supernumerary tooth. Some preliminary tooth movement may be required to create space for the displaced tooth before a band, or better still a bonded bracket, is placed. A new removable appliance is then constructed. This carries a spring which is designed to engage the gingival surface of the bracket and apply occlusal traction.

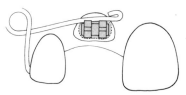

A bracket, bonded onto the enamel of an uncovered tooth, will allow a spring in 0.6 mm wire to move the tooth occlusally.

Retention

When the occlusal level is reached it is usually necessary to retain the tooth in the corrected position. Such retention may be built into any future appliance or may be achieved by passifying the existing appliance.

Rotation

A single rotated tooth in a patient with an otherwise acceptable occlusion may be rotated with a 'whip' where there is adequate space available. Three components are involved:

1 An Attachment to the Tooth

Either a Begg or edgewise bracket may be used, cemented via a single band or bonded directly to the tooth. We find the edgewise bracket most useful.

2 A Sectional Wire

A sectional wire or whip is attached at one end to the bracket on the tooth while the other is hooked to a suitable site on the removable appliance. Whatever design is used provision must be made to avoid its rotating on its long axis. If an

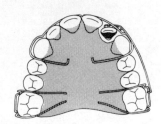

A whip constructed in rectangular wire will not rotate within the bracket slot. The incorporation of coils will allow a light force to be delivered for the correction of a rotation.

Where an incisor has a disto-labial rotation the whip can engage onto the bridge of a molar or premolar clasp. In the case of a mesio-labial rotation the whip would engage the labial wire.

edgewise bracket is used the whip can be made of rectangular or square wire so that it cannot rotate within the bracket slot. Wires which are relatively inflexible should incorporate suitable coils to reduce the stiffness.

3 The Removable Appliance

The appliance will require clasps for retention and will need extra clasps or a labial bow to engage the hook of the whip. For mesio-labial rotations a plain Hawley type bow will serve well. For disto-labial rotations it may be impossible to construct an adequate length of whip to engage the labial bow. The site of engagement may need to be the bridge of clasp on a premolar or molar.

Simple rotations may be corrected in this way, and even over-corrected to some extent. Uprighting of the long axis is less successful although theoretically possible. The difficulty is that the necessary activation will tend to extrude the tooth. The whip itself provides no labio-lingual control, though a single rooted tooth is unlikely to move far. Judicious adjustment of the labial bow will help to control this aspect of tooth movement.

Usually only single teeth should be treated in this way. It may be possible to correct the rotation of two teeth, but only providing that true reciprocal anchorage applies. Thus two central, or two lateral incisors which are similarly mesio-labially rotated may be aligned with crossed 'whips' controlled by the labial bow of the removable appliance. Any other combinations or dissimilar rotations undoubtedly require full banded techniques.

Retention

Rotated teeth are notoriously liable to relapse after treatment. This will be especially so after simple treatment with a whip. In full banded therapy rotations are corrected early, then retained with the bands while the remainder of the treatment is completed — perhaps 12 to 18 months later. Simple treatment with the 'whip' is likely to be completed speedily when no other treatment is contemplated, or towards the end of a course of removable appliance therapy. Such a rotation would not have the benefit of a long period of band control. Prevention of relapse is, therefore, most important. The necessary retention may be carried out in several ways:

1. A removable retainer may be constructed with a fitted labial bow encompassing the rotated tooth alone or including one or two of its neighbours. This may be effective for a broad central incisor but is unlikely to be so for a narrower lateral incisor, or the rounded form of an upper canine. Such a retainer may need to be specially constructed for this task.

2. Mesial and distal spurs may be soldered or welded to the band of the treated tooth in such a way as to engage one neighbour on the labial side and the other neighbour on the palatal side. This effectively prevents any relapse and dispenses with the removable appliance.

3. Pinning or bonding the rotated tooth to an adjacent one. Two teeth may be etched on their contacting surfaces and then bonded with a composite or acrylic filling material. Alternatively, a small staple of stainless steel wire may be cemented into suitable cavities drilled into the palatal surfaces of the treated tooth and a neighbour.

4. Whichever method of retention is selected it must be maintained for a year or longer to be effective. The minor surgical procedure of pericision may be carried out to prevent the post-treatment relapse of rotation and thereby much reduce the need for conventional retention. It has been demonstrated that rotational relapse is due in large part to the tension created in the free gingival fibres and not to changes in the deeper fibres of the periodontal ligament. It is a fairly trivial procedure to incise the free gingival fibres by inserting a small blade down the gingival crevice as far as the alveolar crest and moving it round the tooth. Many operators routinely perform this procedure on recently treated rotations.

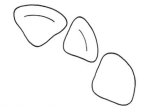

The initial rotation.

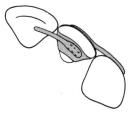

Long term retention may be provided by a single band with welded spurs.

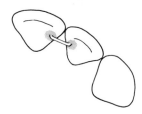

A directly bonded staple of sand-blasted stainless steel wire may be bonded into pits drilled in the palatal surface of neighbouring teeth. This provides unobtrusive long term retention.

CHAPTER 12

'Mutilation Cases'

Malocclusions occur in a wide range of complexity. It is unfortunate that, by the time a patient is first seen by the orthodontist, problems have sometimes been further worsened by the loss or poor state of various teeth.

The term 'mutilation case' is often used to describe such a condition and, for the purpose of classification, the congenital absence and non-eruption of teeth will be considered under the same heading. Mutilation cases present problems for any appliance system. Removable appliances, because of their limited potential, are particularly affected. A case which might have responded well to removable appliance treatment can readily be turned into one demanding a more complex technique. For this reason it is important to avoid unplanned tooth loss, whether in the permanent or deciduous dentition.

In the lower arch in particular, the loss of teeth, whether due to caries, trauma or congenital absence can produce problems beyond the scope of removable appliance therapy. It is important that potential problems are detected early so that any possible interceptive measures may be taken in time to have their best effect.

THE DECIDUOUS DENTITION

In potentially crowded occlusions early loss of deciduous teeth represents one of the commonest dental mutilations. Two types of orthodontic complication may result:

1. Centreline shift;
2. Forward movement of permanent molars.

Centreline Shift

This is commonly associated with the unilateral loss of a deciduous canine. The tooth may either have been extracted, or shed naturally in association with the eruption of a distally placed lateral incisor. The temporary relief of crowding allows the incisors to drift toward the affected side and with continued vertical development the shift occurs bodily.

Such a shift of centreline can present obstacles to successful removable appliance treatment at a later stage. Although minor corrections of centreline can be carried out and the inevitable tipping masked, if necessary, by grinding, anything more than a millimetre or two is not possible. Even if the centreline shift is aesthetically acceptable the operator may be faced with a choice between bilateral permanent extractions, or an extraction on the crowded side only. The former may provide excess space on the less crowded side; the latter may encourage further shift of the centreline.

It is very important that, as far as possible, the centreline of the teeth should be kept in the midline of the face. If a deciduous first molar or canine is lost early a compensating extraction on the opposite side of the arch should be considered with a view to achieving this.

Forward Movement of Permanent Molars

The early loss of a deciduous molar, especially the second molar, may allow the first permanent molar to drift forward and encroach on space which should have been reserved for the premolars. This may increase the space requirements of later treatment and mean that additional extractions or more complex treatment are required.

Unplanned loss of deciduous molars is obviously best avoided. We would not recommend any rules of thumb about balancing or compensating extractions in other quadrants. A problem is not necessarily easier to treat because it exists in two areas rather than only one.

In the upper arch it is possible, following such a loss, to fit a removable space maintainer and so prevent unwanted forward movement of the permanent molars. The appliance need only be worn at night and, in this respect, it is preferable to a fixed space maintainer since it places less strain on patient co-operation. It is also cheaper. In the lower arch removable appliances are less appropriate to space maintenance and a fixed appliance such as a lingual arch is preferable.

We believe, nevertheless, that space maintainers should be used with caution following the loss of deciduous teeth. The extractions may well have been dictated by a high caries rate which is itself a contra-indication to the long term wear of appliances. If a space maintainer is to achieve anything worthwhile it will usually be required for years rather than months and this wear will be in addition to the normal treatment time.

THE PERMANENT DENTITION

The absence, unplanned loss or non-eruption of permanent teeth may dictate that treatment is necessary in cases which might not otherwise have required it, and that treatment which would have been necessary is made more complex.

Upper Central Incisors

The traumatic loss of an upper central incisor is a problem which frequently confronts the orthodontist. It can be difficult to plan satisfactory treatment for such a situation, but there are two chief alternatives:

1. If the lateral incisor adjacent to the lost central is of a good size, and if it is already drifting into the central incisor space, then it may be possible to consider closing the space by mesial movement of this tooth. Subsequently it can be crowned to resemble a central incisor. Such treatment generally requires bodily movement which is beyond the scope of removable appliances.

2. If the central incisor has been lost recently and space is still adequate, then, particularly in those cases where the lateral incisor is unsuitable for later crowning, the mal-occlusion may be treated on its own merits, as if the incisor were still present. The missing tooth may be temporarily replaced with an artificial one on the removable appliance at least while teeth other than the incisors are being moved. This will improve the appearance of the patient, and act as a space maintainer. It is more difficult, however, to maintain the space of the missing tooth during the alignment of irregular incisors, or particularly during the reduction of an overjet. Wire spurs must be incorporated to hold the space and, during tooth movement, these wires may cause friction, or trauma to the gingivae.

After orthodontic retention is completed an eventual restoration for the missing tooth can be considered. This may take the form of a specially constructed partial denture or a bridge.

Upper Lateral Incisors

These may be congenitally absent, or malformed so that their extraction is enforced. This may have considerable influence on treatment planning but there are no special considerations with regard to removable appliance treatment.

Lower Incisors

Where there is some tendency to crowding the absence of a lower incisor or its traumatic loss or extraction at an early stage may allow a good alignment of the remaining teeth. The fact that the arch length between the lower canines will have been diminished is of direct relevance to any upper arch treatment because the canine relationship is a useful guide in the assessment of space and progress. It will no longer be sufficient to achieve a Class I relationship in order to reduce an overjet. The upper canines will need to be placed further distally and it may not be possible to obtain a satisfactory buccal occlusion.

Upper Canines

Upper canines are rarely absent but are frequently impacted in the palate in such a way as to necessitate their surgical removal. There are no special considerations in relation to removable appliance therapy. In some cases the position of the canine may be such that it can be moved into the arch.

If the canine is not visible in the mouth it may be surgically uncovered and a hook attached to it, either by means of a band, or alternatively direct bonding. If very little tooth is visible a further alternative is the use of a small cast silver cap incorporating a hook.

A removable appliance can be provided with a cranked palatal finger spring to engage the hook. The incorporation of shallow posterior bite planes will facilitate the movement of the tooth across the lower arch. Such a procedure may be useful even if the final alignment is to be carried out with bands.

An alternative approach for the correction of severely misplaced canines is surgical transplantation. Before this can be considered there must be adequate space for the tooth to be corrected. Removable appliances may be useful in collecting existing space or in moving the buccal teeth distally on the affected side. Such distal movement may be carried out by means of an appliance incorporating a screw and supported by extra oral traction, if necessary after the removal of the upper second molar.

Lower Canines

These are much less commonly misplaced than uppers. Their loss can pose great problems even when fixed appliances are being used and there are no indications for the use of removable appliances.

Premolars

The congenital absence of these teeth is common both in the upper and lower arch. Where there is no tendency to crowding it may be possible to retain the deciduous predecessors. If this is to be worthwhile they should be in good condition, in occlusion, and with no root resorption occurring.

If there is a space requirement it may be possible to use the space from the absent teeth.

Upper Premolars

Space in the upper second premolar position can usually be utilized to align crowding or permit overjet reduction. If space is not plentiful then the additional tooth movement which the retraction of the premolar demands means that extra oral support is more likely to be necessary. Remember that if buccal canine retractors are necessary the canines and first premolars cannot be retracted successively on the same appliance. A separate appliance will be required. If no such space requirement exists the early extraction of the deciduous tooth may be a sensible measure to encourage forward movement of the permanent molars.

Lower Premolars

If any treatment is required it is likely to be beyond the scope of removable appliances. If maximum possible spontaneous movement is to occur then the absence of the teeth must be detected at the earliest moment. If crowding of the incisors exists it may be possible to encourage distal drift of the erupting premolars and canines by early removal of the deciduous canines and molars.

FIRST PERMANENT MOLARS

The biggest contribution to the disease pattern of the permanent teeth comes from the first permanent molars. A
recent survey on childrens' dental health in England and
Wales noted that by the age of 9, half of the first permanent
molars had become diseased and that among 14-year-olds as
many as 20 per cent of first molars had been extracted
because of decay.

Some points about the loss of these teeth are worthy of
consideration. Extraction of a first permanent molar may
give very varying results depending on the age at which the
tooth is removed, the degree of crowding and the relationship with adjacent and opposing teeth.

In general the likely fate of a first molar should be
apparent at 9 or 10 years of age. Loss of a first molar in a
child of this age will frequently permit the second molar
tooth, which would at that time be unerupted, to move
mesially and erupt into contact with the second premolar
or its predecessor. This spontaneous movement varies from
patient to patient and depends on the stage of dental
development rather than the patient's chronological age. The
most favourable stage is that at which the unerupted second
molar can be seen on X-ray to have its crown calcified and to
have commenced root calcification.

If the condition of a first molar is neglected and its poor
prognosis is not detected until a later stage, and particularly
after the second molar has erupted, the situation becomes
less favourable.

Spontaneous movements are always more predictable in
the upper arch where the second molar is usually distally
inclined before it erupts. It can upright onto its apices and
needs only to migrate a small distance forwards. By comparison its fellow in the lower arch has more commonly a
slight mesial inclination and must migrate bodily forwards
through a greater distance. It also has generally less vertical
eruption in which to achieve any improvement.

In the lower arch in particular mesial drifting of the second
molar tooth can be most unsatisfactory. Mesial and lingual
tilting occur, producing an unsatisfactory occlusion and
usually leaving considerable space distal to the second
premolar.

Second molar eruption following first
molar extraction. The upper tooth has
only to tilt forwards a short distance to
close the space. The lower would have to
move bodily through a greater distance.

Removal of the lower first molar may have unfortunate effects.

Although some spacing of the premolars may occur, it makes little contribution to the alignment of crowded lower incisor teeth. A further complication can arise when a lower first molar has been removed and the upper first molar is left *in situ*. Where there has been a Class I molar relationship the upper first molar can over-erupt into the lower extraction space. The lower second molar is prevented from drifting mesially because its mesial surface contacts the distal surface of the upper molar.

For these reasons it is important that, in cases where the first molars may be at risk, an orthodontic diagnosis and treatment plan is carried out early. Preferably before the age of 10 years.

The action to be taken will depend on the nature of the malocclusion and the quality of the teeth. In general, where the first molar tooth is of doubtful prognosis its removal should be considered at this stage. When a lower first molar has to be removed in this way the extraction of the upper first molar should also be considered, especially if the occlusal relationship is such as to permit its over-eruption.

A problem arises when treatment is to be carried out in the upper arch and it is hoped to make use of the first molar space. It may then be useful to preserve the upper first molar, if necessary by a temporary restoration, at least until the second molar has erupted and can be clasped. If this is not done then the second molar will erupt well forward and the valuable space will be lost. In some cases where crowding is severe it may still be sensible to remove upper and lower first molars at the same time and allow space closure to occur. Later, when the permanent dentition is established the case must be reassessed and it may be possible to justify extractions (most probably first premolars) from the upper arch. This may be particularly useful when there is upper premolar crowding, perhaps as a result of forward movement of the first molars following early loss of deciduous molars. A contra-indication might be displacement of the crowded second premolar palatally.

If crowding is not severe enough to demand the loss of four upper teeth then the early loss of upper first molars may leave a minimal malocclusion which may be treated by the use of extral oral force as the permanent dentition is being established.

100

Removable Appliance Therapy when Upper First Molar Space is to be Utilized

In a malocclusion where a lower first molar has been extracted and the upper tooth temporarily preserved as a space maintainer it is wise to wait until upper second molars are fully erupted before commencing treatment. This is necessary not only to use the full extraction space but also to facilitate the placing of retaining clasps on the upper appliance. Even so, the use of upper second molars for retention does give rise to a number of difficulties:

Eruption Dates

The commencement of treatment frequently has to be delayed, sometimes for several years, while the second molars erupt. Apart from any dental or psychological disadvantages this may mean that treatment is more likely to conflict with schooling at an important stage.

The Teeth to be Clasped are Further Back in the Mouth

This has various effects:

1. *Extra care must be taken with the impression.* It is very easy to find that the impression has not extended fully around the second molars.

2. *The appliance will be longer.* This makes stability more of a problem. Anterior retention will be even more important if the appliance is to remain in place. The addition of extra oral traction is complicated by the need for a longer inner arch on the face bow.

3. *The space produced is further back in the mouth.* This means that more tooth movement must be carried out. Treatment is likely to take longer and there is more opportunity for anchorage to be lost.

4. *There is poorer resistance to anchorage slip.* The large contribution of the first molars to the anchorage is no longer present. It is more likely that extra oral support will be needed.

101

The Second Molars Give Poorer Retention

1. *The shape of the crown is more conical.* This means that undercut is less readily available. The palatal surface in particular tends to be sloping and the fit of the acrylic offers less resistance to the grip of the arrowheads.

2. *The state of eruption.* There may be incomplete eruption of the second molars. It is common to find that even when these teeth are fully in occlusion they still have short clinical crowns.

The Clinical Approach

It must be accepted that treatment after the removal of upper first molars is likely to require more appliances than would be necessary if first premolars were to be extracted. Two alternatives are possible:

1. If Space is Short

The appliance should be constructed with Adams' clasps on upper second molars. Additional clasps will be necessary further forward. Sometimes, if the incisors are proclined, it may be possible to clasp the central incisors. The premolars can then be retracted with palatal finger springs. If the canines are in the line of the arch then they can also be retracted with finger springs but otherwise the acrylic can be cut away so that they can drop into line as space is made. If retention is difficult to obtain on the incisors then it is possible to clasp the canines or the first premolars. In either case it will be necessary to use further appliances if there is an overjet to be reduced. Remember that if this is to be done then each appliance must be designed to maintain the improvement which the previous appliance has achieved. Clasps or stops may have to be placed on first premolars before going on to retract the canines. Extra oral force may be required throughout to support the appliance.

2. If There is No Space Shortage

The upper first molars should be extracted and the patient kept under close observation for a period of a few weeks. The second molars will usually move mesially during this period and erupt further to become more easily claspable.

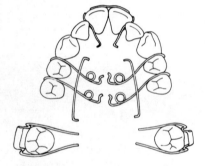

The wirework of an appliance to retract premolars following upper first molar extractions. In this case second molars are fully erupted.

An impression can then be taken for the first appliance, but it is important that the appliance is fitted soon after the impression, and certainly in not more than 7 to 10 days. If this is not done then continued mesial movement of the second molars may make it impossible to fit the newly constructed appliance. This point should be made clear to the patient and parent so that missed appointments can be avoided.

Although second molars which have drifted mesially in this manner may offer better retention it will still be necessary to clasp teeth further forward in the arch as described in the previous section. The details of such clasping will, of course, depend on the precise arrangement of the teeth in an individual case. Palatal finger springs can be used to move the premolars distally. Extra oral support may still be required despite the fact that the second molars were allowed to come forward at the start. Remember that anchorage loss during the retraction of buccal teeth with a removable appliance will produce proclination of the incisors which will subsequently have to be retracted. Such 'round tripping' rarely makes good sense with any appliance system.

Occasionally it is necessary to commence treatment at an earlier stage than this if enforced extraction of the first molars has to be carried out before the second molars have erupted. If this is the case then there may be problems. It is frequently difficult to obtain sufficient retention while leaving the necessary teeth free to move. Treatment may demand the use of consecutive appliances in the following manner:

1. Fit an appliance carrying Adams' clasps on the upper first premolars and a clasp of some type on the central incisors. Palatal finger springs can be provided to move upper second premolars into a better than Class I relationship with the lower arch.

2. A second appliance can be provided with Adams' clasps on the newly moved upper second premolars together with the central incisors. Palatal springs can be used to move back upper first premolars and subsequently upper canines, provided the latter are not buccally placed.

3. Finally a third appliance can be used carrying double Adams' clasps on the premolars on each side, together with stops mesial to the canines and a suitable labial bow to retract and/or align the anterior teeth.

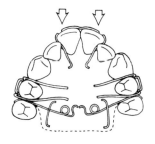

A possible approach where upper first molars have to be lost before second molar eruption. This treatment would need to be started immediately after the extractions. Extra oral force must be applied anteriorly.

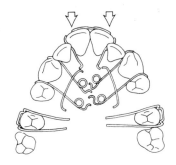

The second appliance, the newly moved second premolars are clasped. Once again extra oral force is necessary.

This type of treatment plan can become complicated and laborious and it may be better to consider alternative means of treatment such as functional appliances, or fixed appliances.

The 'En-Masse' Appliance

A further alternative is to employ an extra oral force directly to effect the distal movement of the buccal teeth. This may be achieved by the use of the 'En-Masse' appliance. This is designed with retentive clasps on four teeth — canines and second premolars when alignment permits this — and moves the buccal teeth distally in one group, hence the name. Midline expansion can be provided by means of a screw or Coffin spring. Provision for the attachment of the face bow is also required. Once the premolars and canines are in better than a Class I relationship to the lower arch then treatment may proceed along conventional lines to reduce the overjet or align the incisors.

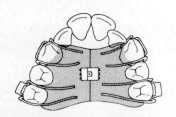

An alternative answer to the problem. An En-Masse appliance using extra oral force to move premolars and canines distally. A midline screw is used to increase arch width as movement progresses.

CHAPTER 13

Treatment of Adult Patients

It is often said that orthodontic treatment is much slower in older patients. Indeed patients in their later teens who ask about treatment are frequently put off by dental surgeons and told that they are 'too late'.

In fact a good deal of orthodontic treatment is possible even in an adult patient but there are important considerations before embarking on this.

The differences between the adult and child patient may be considered under three headings:

       1. Pathological;
       2. Physiological;
       3. Psychological.

PATHOLOGICAL

An older patient is likely to have experienced more pathology than a young one. Caries should be less active but the periodontal condition is usually worse. Teeth of doubtful prognosis will obviously affect treatment and a poor periodontal condition is usually a contra-indication.

Loss of Teeth

Unplanned loss of teeth may present several problems.

Retention

The choice of teeth for clasping may be reduced so that the appliance cannot be adequately supported in such a way that movement can be carried out.

Spacing

Space may be present but in a site where it can only be used after a prolonged period of tooth movement (e.g. residual space from the loss of an upper first molar and shortage of space for an outstanding upper central incisor). Partial closure of space from earlier enforced extractions may have left the patient in a situation where there is too little space for the desired tooth movement but where further extractions are undesirable and would produce excess space.

Spontaneous Tooth Movements

Following unplanned extractions undesirable tooth movements may have occurred. Over-eruption of opposing teeth may cause cuspal locking which will prevent movement. Tilting and rotation of neighbouring teeth may make clasping difficult and interfere with movement.

PHYSIOLOGICAL

The physiological difference between a child and an adult is that the latter is no longer growing. The face is not lengthening and movements which are assisted by growth become more difficult. The age at which an orthodontic patient should be defined as an adult is very variable and, particularly in girls, growth may almost have stopped before the mid-teens.

Bite Opening

The wearing of an appliance incorporating an anterior bite plane will prop the posterior teeth apart. In the growing child these teeth erupt into occlusion so that later, if the appliance is removed, an incomplete overbite can be demonstrated. An adult usually finds the bite plane more difficult to tolerate and, even when it is worn well, bite opening occurs only with difficulty. Similarly the use of posterior bite planes to gag the bite temporarily open to facilitate particular tooth movements is less well tolerated.

Eruption of Teeth

Eruption of buried teeth occurs much less readily in an adult even if space is created and it is sensible to be cautious in one's expectations. Similarly, residual space closes less readily once growth has ceased.

The normal procedures of passive eruption and attrition may have been going on for several years in an adult patient. The longer crown length may provide excessive undercut and it will also frequently mean that the model does not need to be trimmed during the construction of Adams' clasps. If anterior teeth have a mesial or distal tilt and have experienced attrition for a number of years in this position then their subsequent correction will leave them with a very unsatisfactory appearance. Considerable grinding may be required at the end of treatment.

It has been pointed out that removable appliances tilt teeth. It is often noted by patients as well as operators that teeth which have been left in a slightly tilted position at the end of treatment in a child (e.g. retracted canines) become less noticeably tilted as growth continues. Although a certain amount of the tilting may have been an optical illusion caused by the bulging of the gingivae it is likely that continuing vertical growth helps to upright the tooth. It is not wise to count on such changes in an adult.

PSYCHOLOGICAL

Patient motivation is extremely important in all forms of orthodontic treatment. A successful result depends on the maintenance of the patient's enthusiasm throughout the course of treatment.

As the treatment plan will frequently involve extractions it is evident that discontinuation before treatment is complete may leave the patient not merely in the original situation but worse than when the orthodontist was first consulted. For this reason it is important before starting treatment to attempt a reasonable assessment of the patient's co-operation with whatever mechanism will be involved.

Children are frequently unconcerned about their malocclusions. Some are eager to have treatment either because they are more dentally aware or because they have been teased at school. A parent is usually enthusiastic and gives a child support and comfort if enthusiasm flags during treatment. It is highly likely that contemporaries will also be receiving orthodontic treatment, perhaps with similar devices, and it is quite the normal thing to see patients in that age group wearing appliances.

With an adult the situation is very different. Some patients have grown to accept their malocclusions and unless treatment is extremely simple may not consider that it is worthwhile. Others may have become increasingly self-conscious about their appearance but although they would dearly love to achieve some improvement the prospect of wearing noticeable appliances is too much for them to face. The adult is more isolated than the child. It is unlikely that contemporaries will be wearing appliances and because it is considered unusual in that age group a patient may have an exaggerated fear that the appearance and any initial effects on speech will be very noticeable to anyone who encounters him. The increased demands of business and social life make this prospect even more worrying. Even an enthusiastic patient will often not have the benefit of a parent to give support and this is why the attitude of a spouse or partner is particularly important. Encouragement or discouragement during a lengthy period of treatment may have a decisive effect on the outcome.

A removable appliance may seem a good choice for adult treatment because it is less visible than a fixed one but this is often not the case. The fact that an adult may take longer to adapt to the bulk of the acrylic and that the appliance is removable, often tempts the wearer to take out the appliance perhaps for social evenings, for meals, and sometimes at work. This is a very sure beginning on the downhill path towards failure. Some patients recognize their weaknesses and ask for an appliance which they cannot remove.

General Principles

With the exception of points which have been made in this chapter the mechanical details of tooth movement are the same in the adult as in the child. The following general rules should be observed:

1. *Keep treatment simple.*
2. *Make the patient talk you into providing treatment.* Never persuade a patient to have treatment. It is a good plan to avoid the possibility of a patient being swayed by a surge of enthusiasm at the outset. Advise him to go away and think about possible treatment before coming to a decision.
3. *Do not promise too much.* A removable appliance will not carry out the precise tooth movements which a fixed appliance can achieve. Make sure at the outset that the patient realizes that his result will be an improvement on the original situation rather than a perfect occlusion.
4. *Paint the picture a little blacker than you expect.* It is better to over-estimate on the length of treatment time and how visible the appliance will be. A patient who finds that

things are not as bad as he had imagined will be far happier than one who thinks he has been deceived.

5. *Fit an appliance before carrying out extractions.* This is particularly important especially if bite opening is required. If the appliance is well tolerated over a month or 6 weeks then extractions can go ahead.

6. *Keep pressures light initially.* This will avoid undue pain, incorrect insertion, anchorage loss and undesired tooth movement. The response to treatment in adults is quite variable but if no movement is occurring then this should be investigated (see Chapter 18). If the tooth is mobile then cuspal lock may be preventing movement and selective grinding of the teeth may be required. (It may also be necessary to grind the teeth as they move into their final position and so produce artificial wear facets which will match the rest of the occlusion.)

7. *Visibility of the appliance.* Naturally one will attempt to make the appliance as unobtrusive as possible. Buccal canine retractors are well tolerated by adults and tend to cause less displacement than palatal finger springs so that an anterior clasp may often not be required. Some operators use latex elastics anteriorly to reduce the overjet. This certainly provides an almost invisible way of carrying out this movement but does produce some problems. Firstly, it is not possible to put selective pressure on one tooth. Secondly, it is easy for the elastic to slide up the teeth and traumatize the gingivae. Thirdly, unless the elastic is replaced by a wire at the end of treatment it is not possible to retain the result and one may finish with the lower incisors biting the upper forwards and so producing excess mobility and prejudicing stability. If an anterior elastic has been used it is a good idea to make a definitive retainer at the end of treatment.

OTHER DENTAL TREATMENT

It should not be overlooked that orthodontics can be of use to adult patients in conjunction with other branches of dentistry.

Prosthodontics

When a partial denture is being planned it is sometimes evident that the spacing is inconveniently situated. There may be insufficient space to accommodate a normal sized replacement tooth due to drifting of the adjacent teeth. It may be a simple matter to increase this space with a removable appliance and thereby construct a more satisfactory prosthesis. Similarly simple tooth movements may facilitate the construction of a fixed bridge.

Periodontics

In the case of patients who have experienced drifting and spacing of teeth as a result of periodontal disease, simple orthodontic treatment can often be undertaken in association with periodontal therapy to restore appearance. Long term or even indefinite retention will usually be required in such cases.

Surgery

Combined orthodontic and surgical treatment may be indicated.

Prior to minor surgery such as the transplantation of a tooth, treatment may be carried out to create the necessary space.

Prior to major surgery to correct the jaw relationship, some local tooth movements may be carried out to permit the establishment of a good occlusion in the post-operative position. Such treatment commonly involves simple arch alignments or arch expansion.

CHAPTER 14

Treatment of Class I
Malocclusions

Angle classified malocclusions on the basis of the antero-posterior relationship of the first permanent molar teeth. This classification has largely fallen into disuse and is now reserved for the relationship of individual molar teeth. Ballard classified malocclusions on the basis of incisor relationship. Class I relationship exists when the lower incisal edges occlude with the middle third of the palatal surfaces of the upper incisors. This system is open to some of the objections raised to that of Angle, namely that local tooth displacements may create a local relationship which is at variance with the underlying malocclusion.

In a Class I case the occlusion and underlying skeletal pattern are essentially normal in the antero-posterior plane. This normality presents the only constant clinical feature of a Class I malocclusion but many local discrepancies of tooth position and occlusion may be superimposed. Class I malocclusions, therefore, include a very wide range of orthodontic problems.

CLINICAL FEATURES

1. Lateral and vertical skeletal variations;
2. Spacing;
3. Crowding;
4. Local dental problems.

Any of the above features may not only be associated with Class I malocclusions but may be found frequently in any other malocclusion.

TREATMENT

Skeletal Variations
Although the skeletal pattern will by definition be normal in the antero-posterior plane, there may be abnormalities in arch width and vertical relationship:

111

Lateral Arch Discrepancies

Unilateral crossbite. This malocclusion is generally associated with a lateral mandibular displacement in which case the outlook for treatment is favourable. Arch expansion will usually effect the necessary dento-alveolar correction, see Chapter 5. Expansion may be carried out with a removable appliance incorporating adequate retention, preferably with four Adams' clasps on premolar and molar teeth. The active expansion may be carried out by a midline screw or a Coffin spring.

Bilateral crossbite. This malocclusion is rarely associated with mandibular displacement and treatment is usually not indicated. Even in a case where treatment is required it would be beyond the scope of removable appliance therapy.

Total buccal occlusion. The correction of an individual tooth in buccal occlusion may be straightforward. The correction of a buccal occlusion affecting several teeth, either unilaterally or bilaterally may be most difficult and is not appropriate to removable appliance therapy.

Vertical Arch Discrepancies

Open bite. This may be due to skeletal factors or may be an acquired feature of the dentition:

1. *Dento-alveolar anterior open bite.* This acquired malocclusion is a very common one and is usually associated with a thumb or finger sucking habit. Providing the habit ceases while the patient is still relatively young, there is a good prospect for spontaneous resolution. If the habit persists into adolescence then it may be wise to consider appliance therapy designed to assist the patient in abandoning the habit. A suitable appliance could carry Adams' clasps and a 'hayrake' which should effectively interfere with the sucking habit. Alternatively, a passive oral screen may be useful for the patient who only sucks a finger or thumb at night-time.

2. *Skeletal anterior open bite.* This is due to an underlying vertical discrepancy and does not readily respond to orthodontic treatment.

3. *Increased incisor overbite.* Since Class I case is normal antero-posteriorly, there should be an incisal contact which will prevent over-eruption. A deep overbite is normally

112

associated with a Class II or Class III malocclusion.

SPACING

In Britain generalized spacing is comparatively rare. This is fortunate because it can provide a difficult problem for any appliance system.

CROWDING

Crowding of the permanent dentition is probably the commonest indication for orthodontic treatment. It presents in a continuous spectrum of severity from minimal crowding to most severe. Classifications are arbitrary but may be related to the form of treatment selected. There are two alternative methods of dealing with crowding; the first is by extraction of teeth from within the arch. The second method is by distal movement of the buccal segments.

TREATMENT OF CROWDING BY EXTRACTION FROM WITHIN THE ARCH

Tooth loss must be correctly planned if a satisfactory result is to be achieved without undue residual spacing. Tooth alignment may be brought about with appliances or by spontaneous movement. Whatever the mechanism there are certain factors which must be assessed when extractions are being planned:

Molar Relationship

This is an important consideration in treatment planning. We have pointed out that in Class I malocclusions the molar relationship need not necessarily be Class I since such local factors as early loss of deciduous teeth may produce mesial movement of permanent molars.

Class I Molar Relationship

If the molar relationship is Class I, the upper and lower centre lines are co-incident and there are no marked abnormalities of tooth size, then an extraction from each quadrant is likely to be required to relieve crowding. Although, on occasion, any tooth from within the arch may be extracted, the teeth of choice are the upper and lower first premolars. These extractions not only provide the required space to align the upper and lower arches, but also ensure that any residual spacing at the end of active treatment will be equal

113

in opposing quadrants. This should assist spontaneous space closure at the end of retention.

Class II Molar Relationship

Variations in the molar relationship may dictate a modification of the treatment plan. When a full Class II molar relationship is present with crowding only in the upper arch, lower extractions are not required. The aim of treatment is to provide a well aligned upper arch, maintain a good alignment in the lower and finish with a Class II molar relationship with no upper residual spacing.

Intermediate Molar Relationships

Not all malocclusions will fall neatly into the categories outlined above. The molar relationship may be half a unit Class II with the teeth meeting cusp to cusp. This situation occurs commonly and may complicate the choice of extractions. Various options are available:

1. Where there is no lower arch crowding it is possible to extract in the upper arch only. This should encourage the molar relationship to change from partial Class II to a full Class II.
2. When lower crowding is present, upper and lower premolars must be extracted.

If a Class I molar relationship is to be achieved at the end of treatment, it will be necessary for the lower molars to drift mesially to a greater extent than the uppers.

This may be encouraged by extraction of the lower premolars at an earlier stage than the upper. Such an approach will often be appropriate as the later eruption of the upper canines means that upper treatment must be delayed.

In some cases the wearing of an upper appliance will prevent mesial movement of the molars and may be all that is required.

In a few cases it may be necessary to carry out slight distal movement of the upper molars by extra oral force to achieve a Class I molar relationship, from which concurrent space closure may later occur in the two arches.

Asymmetry

Crowding is not always symmetrical. Early loss of deciduous molars may occur unilaterally and permit forward movement

114

of the permanent molars on the affected side only. Similarly, early loss may be associated with a shift of centreline to the affected side.

Provided that the centrelines are approximately correct, each side may be dealt with on its own merits. For example in a particular case it may be possible to extract bilaterally in the upper and unilaterally in the lower arch.

When the centrelines are displaced it may still be possible to consider each side on its merits, but unilateral extraction on the crowded side may lead to further shift of the centreline, while bilateral extractions may leave excess space on the less crowded side.

One solution in a younger patient is to extract a tooth from the uncrowded side, in the hope of some centreline correction, and follow this by an extraction on the crowded side at a later date.

These difficulties and their various solutions may be applied to either or both arches. Wherever possible it is wise to preserve the integrity of the centreline relationship if at all possible and due attention should be paid to this factor in the management of mixed dentitions.

Where no satisfactory solution can be seen it may be necessary to consider the use of a fixed appliance in one or both arches in order to control spaces or centrelines. Some cuspal grinding may be helpful to permit occlusal relationship between Class I or Class II. Remember that spontaneous space closure occurs most effectively in the younger actively growing patient. Treatment planning should be carried out before the permanent dentition is established.

Tooth Size

In some cases particular teeth may be of abnormal size. For example an upper lateral may be small and peg-shaped. Despite a correct centreline and molar relationship, residual spacing is inevitable if upper and lower premolars are extracted.

Even where tooth sizes are normal, the removal of different teeth from opposing quadrants may cause problems. Local tooth displacements may dictate the extraction of teeth other than premolars, which will provide differing spaces in each arch. An example is provided by the extraction of an upper canine and a lower first premolar. This will provide unequal spaces and therefore leave residual upper space.

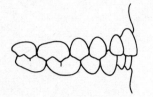

An upper canine and lower first premolar have been extracted. The cuspal interdigitation prevents spontaneous closure of the residual upper space.

This particular example also illustrates a further problem in that non-matching extractions may limit desired spontaneous tooth movements.

APPLIANCE THERAPY FOLLOWING EXTRACTIONS

While some cases may be treated by extraction alone, many will require some appliance therapy in the form of space maintenance or local tooth movements.

Space Maintenance

The need for space maintainance provides a very common indication for removable appliance therapy. A space-maintainer is simple in design, easy to wear and in most cases is effective if worn at night only. It puts no strain on tooth quality and little strain on the patient's co-operation. Only infrequent supervision is required.

Indications for Space Maintenance

A space-maintainer should permit desired spontaneous movements and prevent unwanted tooth movements. In cases where active tooth movement will eventually be required, an appliance may be fitted inactive as a space-maintainer while the necessary teeth erupt. At this stage it may be worn full-time and the springs activated.

Premolar Extractions

First premolars are the teeth most often extracted for the relief of crowding. The upper first premolar usually erupts before the canine and its removal will often allow the canine into a good position without intervention. A simple space-maintainer will prevent forward movement of the buccal teeth, while this occurs. Second premolars are less often extracted but where they are congenitally absent and there is crowding elsewhere, space maintenance may be advisable to preserve the space for later tooth movements.

TREATMENT OF CROWDING BY
DISTAL MOVEMENT OF BUCCAL TEETH

A degree of distal movement of upper buccal teeth may be carried out by use of extra oral forces. In the lower arch this is a much more difficult tooth movement. In a situation where the lower arch can be accepted and the upper arch is only slightly crowded this approach may, therefore, provide a satisfactory solution, particularly if the problem occurs on one side only. The extra oral force may be applied in any of the methods described in Chapters 5 and 16.

LOCAL DENTAL PROBLEMS

Almost any congenital or acquired tooth irregularity could be considered under this heading. It is important that the operator should assess the dentition as a whole and formulate a proper treatment plan rather than simply treat the local irregularity when it is first noticed. Providing the required tooth movements fall within the scope of removable appliance therapy the appliances described elsewhere in this book should serve the purpose.

CHAPTER 15

Treatment of Class II, division 1 Malocclusions

The Class II, division 1 malocclusion is the most common single indication for the use of removable appliances. It is essential that cases of this type are carefully selected. Removable appliances are not suited to the treatment of severe Class II, division 1 malocclusions, particularly those with significant Class II skeletal patterns.

CASE SELECTION

A suitable case should demonstrate the following clinical features:

1. *An increase in overjet of modest degree which is due more to proclination of the upper incisors than to bodily forward position.* 'Upright' upper incisors which are normally inclined can only be tilted a few degrees lingually before becoming unattractively retroclined and making too high an inter-incisal angle for a satisfactory anterior occlusion. Conversely, proclined incisors may be tilted much further lingually before this occurs. Assessment of the underlying nature of the overjet is thus of as much importance as its magnitude.

2. *Individual tooth position should be such that a removable appliance can cope with required tooth movements.* Remember that apical malpositions, rotations, or unfavourably inclined canines are contra-indications.

3. *The lower arch should respond to simple treatment or should require no treatment.* A satisfactory lower arch may be left untreated, or treated by extractions alone where the degree of crowding and tooth inclination makes this possible. Lower fixed appliance therapy may be carried out, although many operators would consider this an indication to use fixed appliances in both arches.

SPACE REQUIREMENTS

Careful assessment of the degree of crowding or spacing must be made, as described in Chapter 6.

The lower arch may require extractions for relief of crowding. The upper arch may also need space to relieve the crowding and in addition space to accommodate the anterior teeth as the overjet is reduced.

CASE ASSESSMENT

We have already described the type of incisor relationship which will respond to removable appliance treatment. It should be remembered that a wide variety of Class II, division 1 malocclusions can occur with such a relationship, and the other features of these malocclusions will determine the detailed treatment plan.

Upper Arch with Adequate Space

In a small proportion of Class II, division 1 cases the molar teeth may be Class I, the lower arch uncrowded and the increased overjet due to proclined and spaced upper anterior teeth. There may or may not be an associated increase in overbite. It is possible to carry out treatment using upper removable appliances without extractions. Extra oral support may be required to prevent anchorage loss.

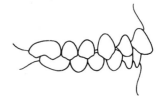

The lower arch is well aligned, the molars are Class I and there is upper arch spacing.

Upper Arch with Minimal Space Requirement

This type may demonstrate a satisfactory lower arch, but there will be some forward displacement of one or both upper buccal segments. The space shortage will present either in the form of an increased overjet or as a combination of a mild overjet with some irregularity. Treatment may involve the use of extra oral force to correct the molar relationship to Class I, followed by removable appliances to reduce the overjet and align the anterior teeth. The correction of the molar relationship may be aided by extraction of the upper second molars. Where the crowding is unilateral a suitable screw appliance supported by extra oral force may be used.

This approach is similar to that which would be used in a Class I case with a normal incisor relationship but with crowding of the upper canines due to forward movement of the upper buccal segments.

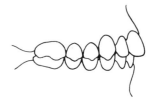

The lower arch is well aligned, but the molar relation is half a unit Class II.

119

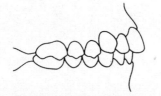

The lower arch is well aligned, but the molar relation is approaching Class II.

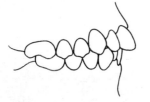

The lower arch is crowded, and because the lower buccal segments are forward the buccal occlusion is Class I.

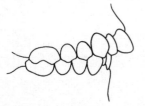

Although the lower arch is crowded with the lower buccal segments forwards, the upper buccal segments are sufficiently forward to produce a Class II molar relationship.

Upper Arch Requiring Extractions

Where the upper arch space requirement is greater but the lower is well aligned it may be necessary to consider upper premolar extractions. An attempt to correct the molars to Class I would require considerable tooth movement, and it is preferable to finish with the molars a full unit Class II. This may be achieved by allowing some anchorage loss during treatment and so permitting forward movement of the upper molars.

Where the molars are Class II at the commencement of treatment, however, extra oral force must be added to prevent any further forward movement during overjet reduction.

Upper and Lower Arch Crowding
with Molars Near Class I

When both arches are crowded and the lower seems likely to respond to extraction therapy then an extraction from each quadrant is necessary. This group probably includes the great majority of Class II, division 1 cases requiring orthodontic treatment. The choice of mechanism will be dictated very much by the molar relationship and degree of crowding. With modest crowding and a Class I molar relationship removable appliances alone may suffice. Where the upper molars are displaced towards Class II extra oral force may be required to prevent their mesial movement. In the lower arch the molars are permitted to move mesially as the anterior teeth align into the extraction spaces and in such circumstances this will aid the correction of the molar relationship.

Upper and Lower Crowding with
Molars Near Class II

This is a severe malocclusion with special difficulties which it is important to recognize. An extraction from each quadrant may provide sufficient lower space but will not do so in the upper. Distal movement of upper molar teeth is necessary in order to gain extra space for overjet reduction and relief of crowding. Where lower crowding is significant mesial movement of the molars can only be permitted to a small degree and will thus make little or no contribution to the correction of the molar relationship. If space is particularly critical in the lower arch then a fixed space-maintainer such as a lingual arch may be indicated. Correction of the molar relationship will require the use of extra oral force. This will be followed by the use of appliances to correct the incisor relationship.

Very Severe Crowding

Some patients present with a degree of upper crowding which dictates the loss of more than two upper teeth. A history of early loss of deciduous teeth is likely. In addition to the extraction of two premolars in the upper arch, it may be necessary to remove a molar from one or both sides. This is likely to complicate the mechanics of treatment so that a decision to use fixed appliances may be wise.

Very rarely a similar circumstance may be present in the lower arch. This would also require tooth movements which dictate fixed appliance control.

A difficult problem, this case demonstrates severe crowding in both arches, and a Class II molar relationship.

Carious First Permanent Molars

Poor quality first permanent molars present special problems in the treatment of Class II, division 1 malocclusions. If they are present when orthodontic treatment is being considered then it may be possible to proceed with their extraction in the lower arch, but to preserve the uppers temporarily until the second molars can be clasped.

Provided that there is not a large space requirement the extraction of upper first molars may be sufficient to correct the malocclusion.

Unfortunately, caries may have occasioned the removal of the first molars before orthodontic treatment is considered. If so then space will have been lost by the mesial migration of second molars so that some space shortage remains. It will be necessary to provide space for the reduction of the overjet. This may be done either by the distal movement of the buccal segments by extra oral force or, alternatively, by the extraction of two premolar teeth in addition to the first molars which have already been lost. The decision must be based on the degree of crowding at the time of presentation together with other factors as, for example, the patient's co-operation with extra oral appliances.

AIMS OF TREATMENT

The aims of treatment should include reduction of the overjet and overbite to within normal limits, alignment of the upper and lower arches and the relief of crowding. The molars should be left in a good Class I or Class II relationship wherever possible. The canines should be in a good Class I relationship. Ideally there should be no space at the end of treatment, but this is frequently impossible to achieve. One should aim to leave only minimal spacing and ideally this should correspond in size and site in opposing arches to encourage spontaneous space closure by mesial drifting.

TREATMENT PLANNING

Before active treatment is commenced full records must be available. These should include study models, X-rays and, perhaps, photographs and lateral skull X-rays where facilities are available. A full complement of developing permanent teeth must be demonstrated, and when second molar extractions are contemplated normal upper third molars must be present on X-ray. Tooth quality must be carefully considered with particular attention to first permanent molars. Remember that lower lingual and upper buccal caries may easily be overlooked. Intra-oral, peri-apical or bitewing films must be taken in cases of doubt.

Once all necessary investigations have been completed and a plan formulated active treatment may begin. An upper impression is taken for the construction of the first removable appliance and an appointment arranged for this to be fitted. Any extractions should ideally be carried out 7 to 10 days before the fitting of the appliance to minimize unwanted spontaneous tooth movements. It is not always possible to arrange things so conveniently and sometimes extractions may unexpectedly have to be postponed. For this reason it is a wise policy to ask the technician to construct the appliance on the intact working model, so that if necessary it may be fitted prior to extractions. An appliance which is fitted before extractions are carried out need only be left out for the duration of the operation.

A CASE ILLUSTRATING TYPICAL TREATMENT

So many variations occur in Class II, division 1 malocclusions that it is difficult to present any one case as being typical. The following example has been composed to demonstrate a number of common features:

Case Assessment

The patient is female, 11 years 4 months of age. Complaining of increase in incisor overjet and crowding affecting upper and lower teeth. The skeletal pattern is mildly Class II, and the overjet 7 mm mainly due to proclination of the upper incisors which lie beyond control of the lower lip.

There is an increased and complete incisor overbite with the lower incisors occluded onto the palatal mucosa just distal to the gingival margin.

The molar relationship is Class I with all buccal segments mesially placed. The upper arch shows slight crowding so that the canines are mesially inclined and on the right side the second premolar is palatally displaced and in crossbite. The incisors are proclined, the centrals more so than the laterals which are themselves lying so that their mesial edges are just obscured behind the distal edges of the central incisors.

The lower arch is crowded with irregularity of the incisors; the centrals being slightly labially displaced when compared with the lateral incisors. The long axes of these teeth are parallel and there is no rotation as seen from the occlusal aspect. The canines are mesially inclined and overlap the distal surfaces of the lateral incisors. The upper and lower centrelines are co-incident.

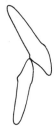

A Class II, division 1 incisor relationship which should respond to removable appliance therapy. Palatal tilting of the upper incisors will reduce the overjet and an anterior bite plane will deal with the overbite.

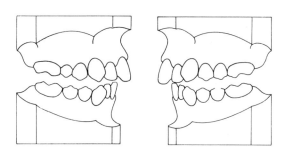

The malocclusion before treatment.

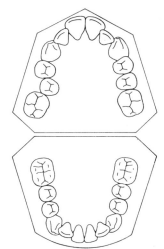

Detailed examination of the dentition shows that the oral hygiene is good. There is no active caries and restorations are only minimal. X-rays demonstrate a normal complement of 28 permanent developing teeth and possible evidence of early calcification of the third molars.

Both the patient and parent are interested in orthodontic treatment and seem likely to co-operate.

Aims of Treatment

a. Relief of crowding.

b. Alignment of the upper and lower labial segments.

c. Reduction of the overjet and overbite to establish a normal incisor relationship.

d. Correction of the crossbite affecting the upper premolar.

e. Maintenance of the Class I molar relationship.

f. Residual extraction spaces to be symmetrical.

Treatment Plan

1. Extract all four first premolar teeth.

2. Fit a removable appliance designed to retract the upper canines into a Class I relationship with the anticipated position of the lower canines. This appliance should also carry a spring to correct the premolar crossbite, and a suitable bite plane to reduce the overbite.

3. Provide a second upper appliance designed to maintain the retracted position of the canines and the reduced incisor overbite, and with a spring to retract and align the incisors.

4. Make provision to retain the new tooth position.

5. Observe the anticipated spontaneous improvement in the lower arch.

Design of the First Appliance

Detailed appliance design may now be carried out with the aid of a study or working model. For this patient a suitable design is illustrated.

Retention

Adams' clasps are used on first molars. In addition some anterior retention is necessary in order to maintain the base plate in contact with the palatal vault. This will contribute towards anchorage and also ensure that the appliance is firmly seated and comfortable. Since the upper incisors are proclined, a fitted labial bow around the central incisors will provide adequate extra retention. The degree of proclination is such as to make the use of an Adams' clasp in this region unsuitable.

Active Components

Canine retraction springs. Whenever possible palatal springs are

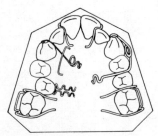

The first appliance, the completed wirework is shown before adding the acrylic.

always to be preferred to buccal springs. In this case, since there is no undue buccal displacement of the upper right canine there is no reason to select other than a palatal spring. On the left side the prominence of the canine will require the use of a buccal spring.

A 'T' spring to correct the premolar crossbite. This useful spring can readily be incorporated on the first appliance so that the premolar can be corrected during canine retraction.

Acrylic Base Plate

Overbite reduction is necessary and, therefore, a flat, anterior bite plane should be incorporated in the base plate.

Fitting the First Removable Appliance

After the usual visual inspection the appliance should be tried in before detailed adjustments are carried out. These may be completed conveniently in the following order:
    a. Adjustment of the retaining clasps.
    b. Correction of the height and horizontal extension of the anterior bite plane.
    c. Activation of the springs.
    d. Trimming of the acrylic to ensure that the anticipated tooth movement is possible.
Finally, the patient and parent must be given instructions in the care of the appliance and an appointment provided in about 4 weeks for the next adjustment.

Management of Treatment Progress

At the second appointment evidence of tooth movement should be present. The canines will have moved distally and the overbite will now be incomplete. If this is not the case, one should strongly suspect that the appliance has not been worn sufficiently. Measurements should be taken using dividers as described in Chapter 9 and recorded on the case-notes. Springs are activated as required. An extra layer of cold cure acrylic can be applied to the anterior bite plane if the molars are once more in occlusion with the appliance in position and further bite opening is desired. Once again, the acrylic should be examined to ensure that it will not impede the distal movement of the canines which is to occur within the next few weeks. Now that the canines have commenced their distal movement it is useful to trim the acrylic around the disto-palatal surfaces of the upper lateral incisors. This will permit these teeth to follow the canines in their movement. Subsequent incisor alignment will thereby be facilitated.

The lower arch should be inspected and measurements taken to confirm that spontaneous distal tilting of the lower canines is commencing.

The patient should then be dismissed for a further appointment when similar adjustments can be made. If progress is uninterrupted then this stage of treatment should be completed in approximately 6 to 8 months. Remember that there is a good deal of individual variation. Interruption caused by holidays, illness and unreported appliance damage may add significantly to the treatment time. At the completion of this stage the following clinical features should be evident:

1. The upper permanent canines have moved distally and approached the mesial surfaces of the second premolars so that the space remaining is approximately 2 to 3 mm. The relationship to the lower canines will be distal of Class I. The lower permanent canines should be making good spontaneous movement but this will not be so rapid as in the upper arch where active appliances have been used.

2. With the appliance removed and the patient occluding in centric relation there should be a reduction in the incisor overbite of the order of 3 mm.

3. The upper lateral incisors should have drifted distally following the movement of the canines. This is brought about by the traction of the trans-septal fibres, and will result in spacing between the central and lateral incisors. The premolar has been moved buccally to correct relationship with the lower arch.

Treatment with the first appliance has been completed.

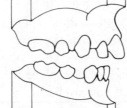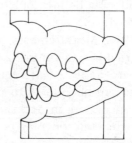

The first stage of orthodontic treatment is now complete. The second appliance can be planned, an impression taken and an appointment given for fitting a week or two later. During this short interval the first appliance should continue to be worn. It is important to emphasize this point as the patient may assume from the dentist's remarks that it has completed its task and is no longer required. Continued wear of the appliance will prevent unwanted spontaneous tooth movements, and it is important that the appliance is made passive so that continued active movements are also prevented. Any such unwanted tooth movements may make the fitting of the second appliance difficult.

Design of the Second Appliance

In addition to carrying out active movements the second appliance has the task of maintaining the treatment progress so far achieved. This means that the canines and premolars must not be allowed to relapse and the overbite reduction must be maintained. A suitable design is illustrated.

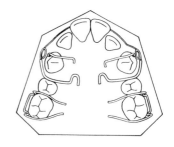

The wirework of the second appliance.

Retentive and Passive Wirework

Adams' clasps. It is not possible to clasp the incisors since they are to be moved. The active labial bow designed to reduce the overjet will, however, contribute to retention. It is permissible, therefore, to design this appliance with only two retaining clasps, on the first molars.

Canine stops. These may be constructed of 0.7 mm soft stainless steel wire and should cross the mesial surfaces thereby leaving the contact points free so that the incisor teeth can be fully retracted.

The Active Component

A Roberts' retractor would carry out the tooth movements adequately.

The Base Plate

This must incorporate an anterior bite plane to prevent any relapse of the incisor overbite. It is passive since no further reduction is required.

Fitting the Second Appliance

Once again this should be inspected and briefly inserted into the mouth to ensure that it is a good fit and comfortable. Thereafter, the necessary adjustments are carried out. Retain-

127

ing clasps are first dealt with, followed by the canine stops as necessary. The anterior bite plane may be trimmed to render it passive. Palatal acrylic should be removed with a suitable bur in such a way as to permit the palatal tilting of the upper incisors.

The labial bow should be activated as described in Chapter 9. The overjet should be measured and recorded in the case notes and the molar relationship inspected to ensure that it remains Class I. The patient may then be dismissed until the next appointment 4 weeks later.

Management of Treatment Progress

At subsequent appointments measurements of the overjet should demonstrate steady reduction and indicate that the patient is wearing the appliance satisfactorily. Further trimming of the palatal acrylic should be carried out in such a way that the anticipated tooth movements occur and yet contact is maintained with the lower anterior teeth to prevent any relapse of the overbite. If treatment progresses satisfactorily then a reduction of the overjet by 1 to 1.5 mm should occur each month. This would make possible the establishment of a normal overjet of approximately 2 mm after 4 to 8 months active treatment. When this stage is being approached and it is evident that the overjet is likely to be fully reduced by the next appointment, the bite plane is completely removed. For a short period, therefore, the lower incisors will have no support to prevent overbite relapse. However, as the initial bite-opening has been successfully achieved and maintained, and the overbite reduction is slightly excessive, full reduction of the overjet can occur before any overbite is re-established.

At this stage it is often possible to remove the canine stops since it is evident that the space between the lateral incisors and the canines is rather greater than required to reduce the overjet fully. This will permit the upper canines to relapse forward slightly and establish a contact with lateral incisors.

Clinical Features at the Completion of Active Treatment

The overjet should be fully reduced with the palatal surface of the upper incisors contacting the labial surface of the lowers. Despite this, overbite is still reduced, with the lower incisors not yet occluding onto the cingulae of the uppers. The upper canines should be in Class I relationship with the lower canines, which by this stage should show considerable spontaneous improvements by their distal drifting. The molar relationship should remain Class I. The extraction spaces distal to the canines should be equal in opposing quadrants and the upper and lower centrelines should remain co-incident.

The appliance can now be made passive and be used as a retainer in the immediate post-treatment phase. When next seen it is likely that the incisor overbite will have increased establishing a normal inter-incisal occlusion, and the upper canines will have moved forwards into contact with the lateral incisors.

Study models may be taken and the patient dismissed for a longer interval of 6 to 8 weeks before the next appointment.

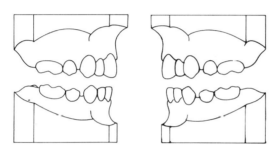

The occlusion at the end of active treatment. Residual space is equal in each quadrant and should close as development continues.

Retention

The patient may be permitted to wear the appliance as a retainer and again dismissed for an extended interval. This phase of retention should continue until the upper anterior teeth feel clinically firm and apparently have a stable relationship with the lower lip. It is difficult to give a clear guidance as to the necessary length of retention other than to say that it should be as long as necessary and as short as possible. In removable appliance orthodontics a conflict arises between the desire to retain a newly created incisor relationship and the necessity of freeing the molar teeth so that spontaneous space closure may occur. In fixed appliance orthodontics it is possible to close the residual extraction spaces in the final phase of treatment and thereafter provide a custom-made removable retainer which may be worn for a considerable period if necessary. In a case such as this, it should be possible to establish an incisor relationship which will quickly become stable within the control of the lower lip. The wisest course in these circumstances, therefore, is to encourage the patient to withdraw the use of the appliance gradually over a period of perhaps 3 to 6 months reducing first from full-time wear to night-time wear and thereafter wearing it for a diminishing number of nights per week until it is evident to the patient and the operator that the incisor relationship remains stable. The appliance can then be discarded and the patient kept under close observation for the next month or two. If it is evident that the treated malocclusion is likely to remain stable the patient may be dismissed for longer intervals.

MODIFICATIONS TO THE BASIC TREATMENT PLAN

The above case has been devised in order to illustrate many of the procedures which are commonly used in the correction of Class II, division 1 malocclusions. Some modification is necessary for other varieties of the malocclusion.

1. *Where no extractions are necessary.* The upper arch spacing is sufficient to reduce the overjet. Canines and premolars are retracted if there is space distal to them, and overbite reduced where indicated. Overjet reduction is carried out in the normal way after any necessary first stage of treatment. If space is only just adequate then it is advisable to add headgear as anchorage reinforcement.

2. *Where upper arch space requirements are minimal.* Upper buccal segments are moved distally with extra oral forces in order to correct the molar relation to Class I. If the third molar teeth are present and of normal crown form then the second permanent molars may be extracted to facilitate this movement. Once a normal buccal occlusion has been established then treatment proceeds as in 1 above, with continued headgear if required.

3. *With an uncrowded lower arch but with upper premolar extractions, treatment follows the illustrated case.* Extra oral traction is not likely to be required as the anchor teeth are to be permitted to move into a full unit Class II occlusion. If the molar teeth occlude in this way at the start of treatment then space is critical and anchorage reinforcement will be necessary.

4. *The severe form of malocclusion with Class II molars and crowding in both arches will require careful assessment and treatment.* Extra oral forces will be needed to correct the molar occlusion to Class I. Four first premolars are re-

moved and appliance therapy as outlined for the example is used. The extra oral support is likely to be required throughout treatment. The lower arch must be carefully observed and a space-maintainer provided if the molars seem likely to drift too far mesially.

5. If more than two upper teeth need to be removed as an elective procedure then special problems with anchorage control and tooth movement are likely. Fixed appliances are the treatment of choice in this instance.

Auxilliary Tooth Movements

In addition to the tooth movements required to move canines distally and reduce the overjet, certain minor tooth movements may be useful.

Bucco-lingual Corrections

Single teeth in crossbite. These have been described earlier. A 'T' spring can often be added to the first appliance to move a palatally displaced second premolar into normal occlusion. If the tooth in crossbite has to be used for clasping then such concurrent movement is not possible. A local crossbite of one first molar can be an inconvenient complication. It is difficult to avoid using an extra appliance for this so that it is best left until the retention stage when a 'T' spring can be used to move it while other teeth are clasped.

Crossbites of several teeth. This, especially when associated with a mandibular displacement, may need to be corrected with an expansion appliance before active canine retraction. If so, then any necessary upper premolar extractions can be carried out to allow some spontaneous drifting of the canines. The expansion appliance acts as a space-maintainer during this period.

Buccally placed canines. When overjet reduction is complete, or nearly so, it frequently becomes apparent that the canines are buccally displaced despite care taken earlier in treatment. This may to some extent be inevitable as the reduction in arch circumference leaves them placed too far buccally. Improvement can be effected by soldering auxilliary springs on to the molar clasps. Canine stops should be removed and acrylic trimmed palatally as necessary.

131

Mesio-distal Tooth Movements

Upper lateral incisors displaced behind centrals. When incisor imbrication is severe then spontaneous distal drifting may not occur sufficiently during canine retraction to facilitate incisor alignment. If this is so then palatal finger springs added to the second appliance will quickly move the lateral incisors to a more favourable position. The addition of these springs does, however, complicate the appliance so that it is wise not to activate the labial bow until this tooth movement is complete. For the same reason the finger springs can be removed as soon as they have carried out their task.

CHAPTER 16

Treatment of Class II, division 2 Malocclusions

Class II, division 2 cases represent a relatively small proportion of all malocclusions and have a great range of severity. Only a few are amenable to removable appliance therapy, and therefore careful assessment is necessary before treatment.

CLINICAL FEATURES

A wide variation of clinical features can be seen in this malocclusion although they may not all be present in every case. The following aspects should be considered:

Overbite

By definition there will be some increase in incisor overbite. This may extend in extreme cases to more than 100 per cent overlap of the lower incisor crowns by the uppers. Trauma to the palatal mucosa by the lower incisors may occur and in very severe cases the upper incisors may traumatize the lower labial mucosa.

Incisor Retroclination

Typically there is retroclination of the upper central incisors. This is very variable and is to some extent related to the degree of overbite. Lower incisor retroclination is a common finding and likewise is associated with the degree of overbite.

Upper Lateral Incisor Position

Classically, both of these teeth are proclined. It is possible, however, to have this feature unilaterally. Often the proclined lateral incisor is rotated mesio-labially. Occasionally a central incisor or canine may be proclined.

133

Skeletal Pattern

Generally this is less noticeably Class II than in the division 1 malocclusion. The severity of the malocclusion is nevertheless related to the underlying basal-bone relationship. There is a reduction in the lower face height which is reflected in the degree of overbite.

Lip Morphology

The lips are competent and the lip line lies high on the crowns of the upper incisors. Classically there is a 'dished-in' appearance of the mid-face with a marked labio-mental fold.

Crowding

Class II, division 2 malocclusions show some upper arch crowding. The upper buccal segments are forward producing a degree of Class II molar relationship and the anterior teeth are retroclined. The arch circumference is thus reduced.

Premolar Occlusion

The upper first premolars are frequently buccally placed and may be in total buccal occlusion. This is occasionally the case with the second premolars.

CASE ASSESSMENT

For convenience of treatment planning, Class II, division 2 malocclusions may be divided into a number of types according to their severity:

A Minimal Malocclusion

The lower arch is well aligned. The buccal segment relationship is half a unit Class II or less and the overbite is only minimally increased. Typically the patient complains of proclined upper lateral incisors. Premolar extractions are best avoided in these cases.

A More Severe Malocclusion

The upper arch crowding is more severe and treatment can be based on upper premolar extractions, this is especially appropriate where the premolars are in buccal occlusion. The situation in the lower arch may vary:

1. There is little or no lower crowding, and because of this the molar relation is likely to be more Class II

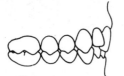

The lower arch is well aligned and the upper buccal segments are only slightly forwards. The overbite increase is minimal.

The upper arch crowding is more severe:

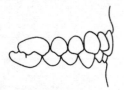

With an uncrowded lower arch the molar relation may be fully Class II.

134

No lower extractions will be required.

2. The lower arch is crowded. Since both upper and lower buccal segments are forward the molar relationship is likely to be more nearly Class I. Lower extractions will be required in addition to those in the upper arch.

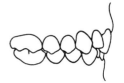

With lower arch crowding the molar relation is only partially Class II.

Most Severe Malocclusion

There is a much increased overbite, which is frequently associated with a severe incisor retroclination. Whether or not extractions are necessary a stable reduction of the overbite will require lingual movement of the root apices to reduce the inter-incisal angle and this can only be carried out with fixed appliances.

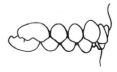

The most severe malocclusion. There is a much increased inter-incisal angle with a deep overbite.

CASE SELECTION

Overbite

We have pointed out that an increased overbite is one of the outstanding clinical features of Class II, division 2 malocclusion. The increase in overbite is associated with an increased inter-incisal angle which prevents the establishment of a normal occlusion between the lower incisal edges and the upper cingula. The incisors are therefore free to continue erupting and to increase their degree of overlap in the vertical plane. Although overbite reduction is sometimes slow, it can be carried out with a bite plane in the same way as for Class II, division 1 malocclusions, but is less likely to remain stable. In Class II, division 1 malocclusions the upper incisors may be tilted lingually into a position where a working contact is achieved with the lowers, thus stabilizing the overbite reduction. In Class II, division 2 malocclusions, by contrast, the upper incisors are already retroclined and a working contact can only be achieved by palatal movement of the upper incisor apices to reduce the inter-incisal angle. This tooth movement is beyond the scope of removable appliances. The significance of this is that removable appliances cannot produce permanent overbite reduction in Class II, division 2 malocclusions and their use should therefore be limited to those cases in which the degree of existing overbite can be accepted.

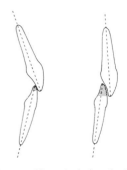

The increased inter-incisal angle allows a deep overbite to occur before tooth contact is established. The Class II, division 2 incisor relationship is illustrated on the right and can be compared with a normal incisor relationship on the left.

The single exception is that it may be helpful to reduce the overbite sufficiently to retract the proclined upper lateral incisors and allow them to establish an occlusion with the

135

lowers. Such minimal reduction should be stable at the end of treatment, if adequate retention is given.

Lower Arch Extractions

It has been held in the past that lower first premolar extractions could lead to lingual 'collapse' of the lower incisors. It has been shown recently that any lingual movement of the lower incisors is small and probably of the order of 1 mm. In most situations this will be insignificant, but in some Class II, division 2 malocclusions it may be critical. Where there is a deep but acceptable overbite this slight degree of lingual movement could increase the inter-incisal angle sufficiently to permit further over-eruption of the incisors and so produce gingival trauma. For this reason lower extractions must be carried out with caution and it is probably desirable to accept a greater degree of crowding in Class II, division 2 than in Class II, division 1 cases.

It has been suggested that a way of avoiding this lingual movement of lower incisors is to carry out any necessary extractions further back in the arch. It seems likely that any extractions in the premolar or first molar region will still permit the slight lingual movement of the lower incisors. Removal of lower second molars may seem the most acceptable alternative to first premolar extraction. This would be appropriate in those cases where the aim of treatment is to prevent further imbrication rather than to treat the existing crowding. Before proceeding with these extractions the presence of third molars of good crown form and inclination must be confirmed radiographically. Oral hygiene must be good and, in particular, first molars must be of excellent quality.

A contra-indication to lower second molar extractions is that third molar eruption is unpredictable.

TREATMENT

Provision of Space

Before the upper incisors can be aligned it will be necessary to provide space in the upper arch. Space can be created in two ways:

1. *Extractions from Within the Arch*

When upper arch crowding is significant and the molar

A critical case, even the slight lower incisor retroclination shown on the left may permit subsequent further eruption of the incisors resulting in gingival trauma.

relationship is half a unit Class II or more, extractions from within the arch can be considered. Unless first molar quality is poor, first or second premolars will usually be the extractions of choice and will provide more than adequate space, so that anchorage preservation is rarely a problem. Where lower crowding exists lower premolar extractions must also be considered.

2. Distal Movement of Upper Buccal Segments (with extraction of second or third molars if required)

The buccal teeth may be moved distally by use of extra oral force as described in Chapter 10. Several methods are available:

1. An En-Masse type of appliance. This should carry clasps on first premolars in addition to first molars. Tubes are soldered to the molar clasps to accept the face bow and provision for midline expansion is made. A screw or Coffin spring may be selected to suit the operator's preference and the technician's skills.

2. Molar bands may be cemented and headgear applied. Once the molars have been moved sufficiently distally a removable appliance can be added to take back the premolars. An anterior bite plane may be incorporated in this appliance if required.

3. A bilateral screw plate may be used. Unless the space shortage is minimal headgear will still be necessary. Once again, an anterior bite plane may be incorporated.

Incisor Alignment

Irrespective of whether space has been achieved by distal movement, or premolar extractions, a removable appliance can now be employed to align the anterior teeth. The necessary tooth movements may often be carried out with a single appliance.

The base plate may require an anterior bite plane to reduce the overbite. The forward position of the upper lateral incisors usually means that palatal finger springs will engage the canines neatly. Buccal springs will combine well with these to correct the lateral incisors when space is available. These springs will themselves offer some retention so that Adams' clasps should only be required on first molars.

Finishing

Because of the element of retroclination of the upper incisors

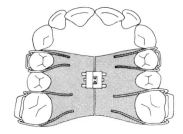

Where the premolar and molar teeth on both sides are in good alignment they may be moved distally *en bloc* with the headgear force applied to a removable appliance.

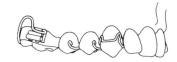

Here the molars have been moved distally using bands and a removable appliance has now been added to move back the premolars.

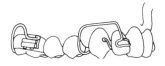

Incisor alignment, a palatal finger spring moves the canine distally. The buccal spring can be activated subsequently to align the lateral incisor and will also act as a stop mesial to the first premolar.

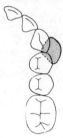

Although the overjet may be normal the presence of an increased overbite means that the necks of the upper incisors are further forward than normal. Similarly the upper canines will also be forward of a Class I relationship.

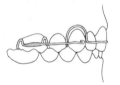

A soldered auxiliary spring added to a retainer to move a slightly outstanding canine palatally.

TOOTH MOVEMENT WITH REMOVABLE APPLIANCES

at the end of treatment, the canines will usually still be forward of a Class I relationship with the lower arch. The canine occlusion will be such that the uppers are buccally placed. Selective grinding and the provision of soldered auxiliary springs as required will improve the appearance. Where extractions have not been carried out within the arch, the buccal teeth will reflect the relationship of the canines and may not interdigitate. Some selective cuspal grinding may be necessary to ensure a stable buccal relationship.

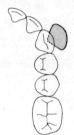

A Class I canine relationship.

A half unit Class II canine relationship. In this position the upper canine is displaced buccally by its contact with the lower.

RETENTION

Many malocclusions which have been treated with removable appliances may be retained by using the final appliance in a passive form. A Class II, division 2 case, however, will often require special attention using a purpose built appliance.

When the anterior alignment is complete the case should be re-assessed. There is no doubt that the proclined lateral incisors are prone to relapse at the end of treatment and it may be necessary to prolong night-time retention until these teeth become firm, when the retention can be gradually withdrawn. A period of at least one year is necessary. Relapse may be related to tension created in the transeptal fibres, particularly when the lateral incisors were originally a little rotated. Slight rotational relapse of these teeth may allow the lower lip to displace them labially.

138

CHAPTER 17

Treatment of Class III Malocclusions

Although Class III cases only represent a small proportion of all malocclusions they include as wide a range of variations as any other group.

CLINICAL FEATURES

Since the nature of the malocclusion will have a direct bearing on the prognosis for removable appliance therapy a thorough examination should be carried out and the following clinical features should be considered:

1. *Skeletal Pattern*

This has great bearing on any other clinical feature and must be looked at in all three planes of space.

2. *Incisor Crossbite*

The recognized principle feature of a Class III malocclusion is the presence of one or more upper incisors in crossbite. Where the underlying skeletal pattern is almost normal, it is unlikely that more than one or two of the incisors will be in lingual occlusion. By contrast a more severe skeletal discrepancy will usually mean that more anterior teeth are in crossbite.

3. *Incisor Overbite*

Incisor teeth which are in crossbite may exhibit any degree of overbite. The extent of this overbite largely reflects vertical skeletal factors, and influences the prognosis for stability.

negativ ovebite.

4. *Incisor Inclination*

This may vary considerably in both arches. When the skeletal pattern is Class I an incisor crossbite can only arise as a result of adverse incisor inclination. With a definite Class III skeletal pattern the incisors will be in crossbite even though they are normally inclined. In some cases with a less marked Class III pattern a crossbite may have arisen as a result of a combination of these two factors.

From time to time a single incisor, perhaps an upper lateral, is displaced bodily into the palate. Such a tooth will require individual assessment before treatment is commenced as the apex may be too far palatally displaced to permit crossbite correction. (F(x)

5. Mandibular Displacement

When an incisor crossbite is present with a positive overbite it is often possible for the patient to occlude with the incisors in an edge to edge position, while the posterior teeth are still out of occlusion. In order to achieve a posterior occlusion the patient displaces the mandible forwards. This is a favourable finding as it demonstrates that the true antero-posterior discrepancy is less severe than first seems apparent. Where there is no incisor contact a forward mandibular displacement will be absent. This situation occurs where there is no overbite or where the severity of the antero-posterior skeletal discrepancy prevents incisor contact.

6. Buccal Crossbite

A Class III malocclusion with a discrepancy in dental bases is likely to have a lack of co-ordination in widths as well as in arch lengths. Crossbite in the buccal segments is a common finding. It may occur unilaterally in association with a mandibular displacement or, less favourably, bilaterally without displacement.

7. Upper Arch Crowding

This is commonly present to some extent and may reflect a small sized upper dental base which is contributing to the skeletal pattern.

8. Lower Arch Crowding

By the nature of Class III malocclusions crowding occurs less frequently in the lower arch. This is particularly so in more severe cases where the lower arch may be noticeably larger than the upper.

140

9. *Growth Effects*

Growing patients who show a Skeletal Class III pattern must be viewed with caution. Such a discrepancy is likely to deteriorate with further growth. This is particularly so in boys, in whom growth ceases later. Simple incisor crossbites on a normal, or nearly normal, skeletal base may appropriately be treated in the early mixed dentition.

More severe malocclusions are best assessed after the pubertal growth spurt and the establishment of the permanent dentition. There is no place for 'orthopaedic' interceptive treatment in Skeletal Class III malocclusions.

CASE ASSESSMENT

The factors referred to above must be considered. Particular attention should be paid to the degree and nature of crowding, the degree of overbite, and the apical position of the lingually displaced teeth. To simplify treatment planning it is convenient to subdivide these malocclusions according to their severity and the nature of the incisor relationship:

1. Class III Incisor Relationship on a Skeletal I Base

The commonest case presenting with lingual occlusion of one or two upper incisors might probably fall within the definition of Class I malocclusion. Because of the mechanical principles of the treatment, however, it is conveniently dealt with as a Class III malocclusion.

2. Class III Incisor Relationship on a Skeletal III Base

The problems of such a case differ from those above only in degree. It is likely that several teeth may be in lingual crossbite, and depending on the nature of the underlying skeletal pattern other factors such as mandibular displacement, inclination of the incisors or degree of overbite may be less favourable. The larger size of the lower arch means that crowding is less likely to be present and lower extractions may not be required.

3. Class III Incisor Relationship with Reduced Overbite

Where there is no overbite, or where an anterior open bite exists there will be no mandibular displacement to eliminate and no possibility of creating an overbite to retain any forward movement of the upper incisors. For the same reason lingual tilting of the lower incisors is unlikely to prove stable.

141

4. Severe Class III Malocclusions

Some malocclusions, either because of the complexity of tooth irregularity or severity of skeletal pattern, will require treatment beyond the scope of removable appliances. Fixed appliances may be needed either alone or in combination with surgery. Removable appliances will only be of service in carrying out minor local tooth movements while the incisor relationship is either accepted or reserved for later surgical correction.

CASE SELECTION

The correction of a Class III incisor relationship may be carried out in a number of ways:
1. The upper incisors may be moved labially.
2. A combination of upper incisor proclination and lower incisor retroclination may be employed.
3. Skeletal surgery may be undertaken with or without the aid of orthodontic treatment.

It would be possible for a patient to wear upper and lower removable appliances at the same time so that reciprocal incisor movements could be carried out. Most orthodontists would, however, prefer to use fixed appliances in these circumstances in order to take advantage of Class III traction. Removable appliances will deal effectively with cases requiring proclination of upper incisors only.

OVERBITE

Because the existence of a positive overbite will stabilize upper incisors which have been moved out of crossbite, it is desirable to finish treatment with adequate vertical incisal overlap. Since removable appliances carry out tilting movements, the forward movement of an upper incisor is invariably associated with some upward movement of the incisal tip. This effect is similar to the swing of a pendulum, the end of which must rise as it moves from the vertical.

Where the original overbite is deep, the tooth will probably finish with a normal overbite after correction. Where overbite is initially within normal limits there will be a reduced overbite, or even a lack of overbite after tooth movement. This reduction in overbite will be even more apparent if the tooth is already proclined before treatment, i.e. if its apex is markedly palatally displaced.

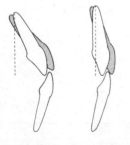

Simple proclination of an upper incisor will inevitably reduce its overbite. This effect is more marked when the apex is palatally displaced.

142

Cases suited to removable appliance treatment should ideally exhibit the following clinical features:

1. There is minimal skeletal discrepancy.

2. A forward mandibular displacement is contributing to the incisor relationship. It should be possible for the patient to reach edge to edge occlusion.

3. The upper and lower arches are well aligned or have irregularities which will respond to local tilting tooth movements.

TREATMENT PLANNING

Crowding

Any space required for incisor correction may be provided in the following ways:

Intrinsic Space

The correction of instanding teeth is unique in that unlike other tooth movements space is created rather than consumed. As incisors are moved forwards they increase the radius of the arch and so provide some useful space. In a situation where the arch appears to be mildly crowded this extra space may be sufficient to permit alignment.

Distal Movement of Buccal Teeth

When proclination alone would provide insufficient space, distal movement of the buccal teeth may be considered. True reciprocal anchorage may well apply in these cases. An appliance which advances the anterior teeth may also move the buccal teeth distally to some extent. An appliance carrying a single screw will advance the upper incisors when the canines are in good alignment with the buccal teeth. If the canines are buccally placed then an appliance carrying bilateral screws may be used to move the buccal teeth distally prior to advancing the incisors.

This provides one of the few examples of a situation where extra oral force may be used with advantage in Class III treatment. Headgear applied to tubes on the molar clasps will assist the distal movement of the posterior teeth. Activation of the screws will maintain the incisors in a forward position. Second molar extractions may be carried out to facilitate these movements.

Extractions

If crowding is more severe space can be provided by extraction of premolar teeth. It may be necessary to carry out other tooth movements prior to incisor correction. For example, canines may be moved distally. Rarely, in cases of severe local irregularities or palatally displaced incisor apices, it may be necessary to extract one or both upper lateral incisors. The lower arch may require balancing extractions but should be considered with discretion where the skeletal discrepancy is great. Space closure in these cases can be disappointing.

Incisor Correction

Once adequate space has been provided, the incisor relationship is corrected with an upper removable appliance carrying suitable springs (described in Chapter 4) to advance the teeth which are in lingual occlusion.

The Base Plate

It is not normally necessary to add posterior bite planes in order to relieve the incisal interference during correction. In most cases tooth movement is permitted by further forward mandibular displacement until it is possible for the patient to avoid edge to edge contact and bring the mandible into occlusion by hinge movement. A simple base plate will, therefore, suffice in all but the few cases which exhibit a very deep reverse overbite. Even in those cases it will not be necessary to separate the posterior teeth sufficiently to eliminate the overbite fully. Posterior bite planes should always be kept as shallow as possible.

Appliance Retention

Springs acting on the palatal surfaces of upper incisors exert a displacing force on the appliance. It is, therefore, essential to have excellent retention of the appliance especially anteriorly. In addition to clasps on first permanent molars one, or preferably two, teeth further forward should be clasped. The site of these clasps depends on the teeth available and on which incisors are to be moved. Occasionally, first deciduous molars or deciduous canines are suitable and in this case 0.6 mm wire is used. In the late mixed dentition when these teeth have been shed or are mobile, then premolars or permanent canines may be utilized. Occasionally an incisor may be clasped provided that it is in normal buccal occlusion. Neglect of this principle of retention is one of the commonest causes of failure.

Springs

Springs may be selected to suit the operator's preference and the needs of the case. Individual 'Z' springs or cranked palatal finger springs may be used. When the appliance is fitted the clasps are adjusted and the springs gently activated. If a spring is merely advanced forwards it may be difficult for the patient to insert the appliance without trapping the spring between the base plate and the incisal edge. Activation of the spring slightly upwards as well as forwards makes for easy insertion. The patient is seen rather more frequently than is required for most appliances, perhaps every 3 weeks. The incisal tip needs only to move through a short distance so that incisor correction should be complete in at most 2 or 3 months.

Retention and Stability

The need for retention will depend upon the degree of overbite. Where this is adequate at the end of treatment no retention will be required once the immediate post-treatment tooth mobility has settled.

In some cases when the overbite is reduced stability may be more doubtful. In such a situation it is a good plan to passify the springs or remove them and replace them with cold cure acrylic. This may be added at the chairside and adjusted by placing the appliance in the mouth before the final set.

The appliance is thus converted to a retainer and may be worn full time at first and subsequently at night until the teeth are perfectly firm before proceeding to gradual withdrawal.

Where there is no overbite after correction it may be useful to overtreat the incisors and maintain this position. The result is that when the retainer is withdrawn the teeth have a chance to erupt slightly and establish some overbite before they can relapse into lingual occlusion.

In cases of deep overbite where posterior bite planes have been required it may be tempting to discard the appliance as soon as the lingual occlusion has been corrected. During

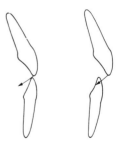

A corrected incisor with reduced overbite will tend to relapse. It is wise to overcorrect the tooth so that there is an opportunity for some overbite to be established.

treatment there will have been some depression of posterior teeth and if the appliance is suddenly abandoned the patient may temporarily have a posterior open bite. In attempting to achieve a posterior occlusion a young patient may posture the mandible forwards and so encourage a return to the original situation. It is safer to continue wear of the appliance after the bite planes have been removed and if necessary removal can be carried out progressively over two visits.

Special Problems with Class III Malocclusions

Treatment Timing

In general a Class III malocclusion should be treated in the established permanent dentition. There are exceptions to this.

Occasionally the anterior teeth erupt into such a position that one or more lower incisors are trapped labially to the uppers while the remaining lower incisors occlude normally. In this situation it may be impossible for the patient to displace the mandible and avoid trauma. If treatment is not provided promptly the affected lower incisors will become progressively mobile and marked recession of the labial gingival margin may occur.

From time to time an upper lateral incisor erupts into lingual occlusion in a crowded upper arch. Extraction of the deciduous canine will provide space for the immediate correction of this tooth. If this is not done at an early stage, then the developing permanent canine will limit tooth movement until a premolar can be extracted and the canine moved distally.

Incisor Intrusion

We have already described the way in which proclination of an upper incisor reduces its overbite. In addition to any normal tilting, the action of the proclining spring on the sloping palatal surface produces an intrusive force, and will further reduce the overbite. Sometimes the reduction in overbite may be quite spectacular, and this may be a particular problem in the case of a lateral incisor which will already have a shorter clinical crown than the central. Correction should be overdone and a short period of retention given while the tooth becomes clinically firm. There is every prospect that the overbite will increase before the incisor has a chance to drop back into lingual occlusion.

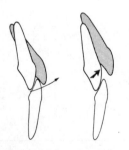

In addition to overbite reduction which might be anticipated as a result of incisor tilting, there may be some intrusion as a result of spring pressure on the sloping cingulum.

If the above method is ineffective a solution is to increase the crown length by adding to the incisal edge with a composite material.

In certain circumstances there may be no prospect of obtaining any overbite at the end of treatment.

Examples are:

1. The alignment of the upper incisors in a severe Class III occlusion where the relationship of the labial segments is to be accepted.

2. The proclination and alignment of upper incisors in a case with an existing anterior open bite.

In such situations very long-term retention will be necessary to ensure that the teeth remain stable and nocturnal wear must be considered over a period of some years.

CHAPTER 18

Failures and Problems

With any appliance system failures can occur and problems may arise during treatment. Removable appliances are no exception and it is important that any difficulty is diagnosed as soon as it occurs so that it may be quickly corrected. Early correction saves valuable clinical time and keeps treatment as short as possible. Prompt detection of inadequate progress will guarantee the operator the respect of a patient who is attempting to conceal his non co-operation.

Failures and problems may present in many different ways and at various times throughout treatment. There may be lack of progress either from the outset or at some stage during treatment. There may be unwanted tooth movement. There may be a complaint by the patient or his parent.

UNSATISFACTORY PROGRESS

There are many possible causes of poor progress. The operator, the technician, or the patient may be at fault. Since it is the operator who selects the cases, plans the treatment and designs and fits the appliances, it is he who must accept the main responsibility. Frequently the orthodontist is asked by an eager parent to provide treatment for a reluctant child. Parental support may be ineffective in persuading the child to wear an appliance which he can readily remove, particularly when he is not under immediate supervision. If treatment has not yet commenced the solution may be to postpone it for a year or two in the hope that the patient, who will by then be more mature, may become eager for something to be done. If treatment has already commenced the orthodontist must discuss the problem with the patient and hope to bring about a change of heart.

Case Selection

Failure to select cases which are within the scope of removable appliance tooth movement is likely to lead to disappointment both to the operator and the patient.

Treatment Planning and Case Management

Correct case selection does not guarantee that the treatment will progress satisfactorily. Faulty appliance design and incorrect management of the appliance or the patient may still give rise to problems:

Appliance Design

An appliance which is bulky or too complex may be difficult to wear. Problems commonly occur when bite planes are excessively thick. Inadequate retention may make it difficult to maintain the appliance comfortably in the mouth.

Appliance Adjustment

Springs which are over active or clasps which are too tight may cause pain to individual teeth. Trauma to soft tissues of the cheek may occur, particularly from buccal springs and labial bows. These must be correctly adjusted to lie comfortably between the alveolus and cheek.

Patient Problems

An appliance may be worn incorrectly by a patient who does not fully understand its action. It is common to find that a patient has inserted the appliance with a palatal finger spring on the distal rather than mesial of a tooth which is to be retracted. A screw may be reversed either because the patient has turned it in the wrong direction or from the wrong side of the base plate. Such difficulties should be prevented by careful explanation to patient and parent at the time of fitting. More particularly the patient should demonstrate that he can insert and remove the appliance before being dismissed with a further appointment.

PROBLEMS WITH PROGRESS — DIAGNOSIS AND REMEDY

When inadequate progress is noted it is tempting to assume that this may be due to an inherent resistance to tooth movement.

149

Although individual variations do occur it should be emphasized that a tooth will move if the correct force is applied for an adequate time and in the absence of obstruction or pathology. Unsatisfactory progress may present in a number of ways:

There Has Been No Change Since the Last Appointment

When progress is assessed at a routine visit measurements may show that no change has occurred although the appliance was activated at the last appointment. If the case has been correctly selected, the treatment plan is sensible and the appliance well designed and constructed then the first suspicion must be that the appliance is not being worn. Parental opinion may be misleading since the astute patient may deceive his parents. Obviously the initial approach is to question the patient directly, but since one cannot rely on an honest answer the clinical signs are important and should be looked for before the patient is questioned.

Useful clinical signs are:

1. The appliance is not worn when the patient enters the surgery. The patient may explain this on the grounds that it was taken out just prior to the appointment either for cleaning or to show the dentist. It is likely that such a patient is not an enthusiastic appliance wearer.

2. Speech is poor. Normal speech should be possible after the appliance has been worn for a few days. If speech is poor with the appliance in position then it is probably receiving, at best, partial wear.

3. The appliance still looks new. An appliance may be still active as though very recently adjusted. The acrylic is shiny and there are no tooth marks from occlusion with the lower teeth and no calculus on the acrylic or the wires.

4. The mouth shows no signs of appliance wear. If the appliance is being worn properly there is usually some reddening of the mucosa under the acrylic compared with the mucosa beyond the area of cover. Frequently there is a well-defined line where the acrylic finishes across the palate. The absence of these signs is almost diagnostic of poor wear.

5. The appliance is a poor fit and difficult to insert. After a period of continuous wear almost any appliance should be clearly a good fit. The retention should be somewhat slackened as a result of normal insertion and removal.

6. The patient is slow and clumsy at appliance insertion and removal. In most cases this indicates a lack of practice as the patient quickly becomes more adept than the operator at inserting his own appliance.

There Has Been Limited Change Since the Last Appointment

In some cases tooth movement may have occurred, but it may be less than anticipated. The appliance is obviously receiving at least some wear. Look particularly for progress on one side but not on the other as this indicates faulty adjustment or obstruction to tooth movement. The failure of the bite to open, even though the canines are moving distally as planned, usually indicates inadequate wear.

Possibles causes of inadequate progress may be:

1. The appliance is only worn part time. This is particularly common in older teenage patients. The appliance is frequently removed for mealtimes which makes overbite reduction disappointing.

2. The appliance is interfering with tooth movement. A tooth may have come into contact with the base plate since the last appointment due to failure to anticipate the movement and trim the acrylic adequately.

3. There is occlusal interference. Cuspal locking by teeth in the opposing jaw may hinder almost any tooth movement. The problem arises particularly in adult patients. The addition of a bite plane to provide temporary relief of cuspal lock may permit normal progress. Alternatively careful cuspal grinding may be all that is required.

4. There is root pathology. Where there is a history of trauma or tooth re-implantation there may be ankylosis. This problem is rare but will totally prevent tooth movement.

5. The appliance has not been adequately activated. The operator may not have adjusted the springs sufficiently or built up the bite plane as required.

6. An unerupted tooth is impeding progress. This difficulty should have been anticipated during case assessment.

7. Headgear is inadequately worn. When headgear is employed directly to move teeth insufficient wear will obviously limit progress.

Undesired Tooth Movements

From time to time unwanted tooth movements may occur. Such movements are likely to be slight if the patient has not missed appointments and the operator exercises due attention. Adverse changes may occur in teeth other than those which are undergoing active movement. The entire dentition should be inspected at each visit so that problems are not overlooked. Common problems are:

1. *Posterior Teeth Move into Crossbite*

This may be brought about during distal movement of buccal segments by failure to increase the inter molar width adequately at the same time. A correctly activated Coffin spring or a properly turned screw will prevent this.

Poorly made clasps may be over enthusiastically adjusted in an attempt to achieve adequate retention and in so doing may move the teeth in a palatal direction. This will occur particularly when only two teeth are clasped and especially if they have sloping palatal surfaces.

2. *Teeth May Move Buccally*

This occurs particularly when canines are being moved distally and can be due to badly sited palatal finger springs or faulty adjustment. In some cases the choice of a buccal rather than a palatal spring would have prevented the buccal movement.

3. *Relapse*

Failure to support recently moved teeth by appropriate stops on a new appliance or by the provision of a suitable retainer may permit some degree of local relapse. The closure of a reduced overbite due to careless adjustment or to absence of a bite plane on a second appliance is a special problem.

4. *Excessive Tilting*

Whenever a tooth is moved by a simple spring some degree of tilting is inevitable. In some cases such tilting will be undesirable. An upper canine which has been retracted may often appear distally tilted. Some of this may be more apparent than real and is due to the heaping up of gingival tissue on the distal aspect of the tooth. Certainly the tilting

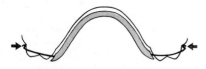

Normal fit of the appliance against the vault of the palate.

Excessive clasp activation may cause the appliance to spring slightly away from the palatal mucosa. If the palatal surfaces of the clasped teeth are sloping, they will be able to move palatally in response to clasp pressure. Repeated activation in a vain effort to improve retention can eventually produce a crossbite.

appears to diminish during the period of retention and afterwards. This improvement may be due to gingival re-modelling or to genuine uprighting of the tooth associated with further downwards and forwards growth of the dento-alveolar complex after treatment.

When upper incisors are retracted to reduce an overjet there is bound to be some tilting. In a case where the incisors are proclined before treatment and the skeletal base is normal this tilting will bring the incisors to a pleasing inclination as the overjet is reduced. If the skeletal pattern is more markedly Class II, then at the end of overjet reduction there will be a degree of incisor retroclination. This must be accepted if treatment has to be carried out with removable appliances. It is wise to make this clear to the patient at the outset to avoid disappointment.

In the more difficult cases where the degree of eventual tilting is likely to be severe treatment should not be attempt-ed with removable appliances.

Partial overjet reduction would be a possible alternative, but although this may give a satisfactory aesthetic improve-ment the result is unlikely to be stable. If such treatment were to be undertaken indefinite retention would be required.

In these two examples the overjet is equal. On the left the upper incisors are proclined and simple tilting will provide an aesthetically pleasing result. On the right a skeletal discrepancy exists. Treatment with removable appliances will inevitably produce unattractive retroclination of the upper incisors.

5. Unwanted Rotations

Sometimes a tooth which is being moved mesially or distally may unexpectedly rotate. This occurs usually when pre-molars or canines are being moved. Such rotations are difficult to predict and prevention is thus a problem. Possible causes are the application of the force too far from the axis of rotation, or the presence of an atypical root shape which may interfere with normal movement. If the rotation is minimal it can be accepted, and provided that it is not retained by subsequent appliances, it may relapse favourably. If the degree of rotation is not acceptable then a fixed appliance will be required.

6. Anchorage Loss

Most tooth retractions which are not aided by extra oral forces will result in a degree of anchorage loss. Except in cases where reciprocal anchorage is being employed to close space this will be undesirable. Proper appliance design and the movement of small numbers of teeth at any one time should preserve anchorage. The avoidance of heavy forces will also help. Unexpected and significant anchorage loss is often associated with failure to wear headgear. The remedy is to ensure that headgear is worn and to passify the active components until the anchorage has been re-gained.

Patient Complaints — Poor Progress

Problems may sometimes come to light as the direct result of a complaint by the patient or parent.

Such a complaint may be unfounded and due to impatience or misunderstanding. In the early stages of treatment, particularly where distal movement of buccal teeth is being carried out prior to incisor alignment, tooth movement may be satisfactory but the patient is unable to see it.

Most complaints by patients are, however, justified. Poor progress will be real and the patient will usually be aware of the cause if there are difficulties with the appliance. In this case corrective measures are usually straightforward.

Some likely complaints are:

1. The initial difficulties with speech and eating have not been overcome. This may be due to a patient's poor tolerance, lack of perseverance or because of inadequate explanation by the operator. Poor adjustment of bite planes is a common underlying cause. Provided that the appliance is satisfactory reassurance may be all that is required.

2. The appliance has been damaged. Fractures of the acrylic or damaged wirework may render the appliance unwearable.

Broken springs will usually need to be remade and processed into the base plate with cold cure acrylic. The original model will make it very much easier to effect a repair. Broken Adams' clasps may be repaired with a spot of solder if they fracture at the arrowhead. If the breakage occurs near the acrylic then part of the clasp may be cut off and treatment continued with some retention from the modified clasp. An appliance which has been provided with three or more clasps at the outset can continue for a short time even where a clasp has to be wholly or partially removed.

Progressive loosening of the appliance or multiple clasp and spring fracture is frequently caused by a patient who habitually 'jiggles' the appliance with the tongue. Such a

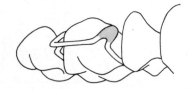

A fractured Adams' clasp repaired by filling in the arrowhead with a spot of solder.

habit should be suspected when the parent, rather than the patient, complains that the appliance is loose. It should be pointed out to the patient that this habit, if continued, will cause repeated breakage and much loss of valuable time to all concerned.

A removable appliance rarely fractures intra-orally. If there is a clean break then it may be possible to repair it speedily with cold cure acrylic. The availability of the working model can simplify any repair. It is wise therefore to have this returned by the technician and kept in the study model box until the appliance is discarded.

3. The appliance has been left out for a time and no longer fits. Illness or accident may provide good reasons for this and so may local pathology such as aphthous ulceration. Occasionally an appliance is left out by a patient who has become concerned by the increased mobility of the teeth being moved. If the period of non-wear has not been more than a few days it may be possible to adjust the appliance to fit so that treatment may continue.

4. Appliance loss. The loss of an appliance may occasionally be justifiable but is more commonly due to carelessness or even to a deliberate act. If the patient reports the loss promptly then a new appliance may be quickly provided before any tooth movements can relapse. Accidental loss is more likely to befall a part-time appliance such as a retainer.

Patient Complaints — Pain and Discomfort

A moderate degree of discomfort is to be expected when any orthodontic appliance is first fitted. During active tooth movement there may be some sensitivity of the teeth. Most patients quickly accept this and come to expect a temporary increase in discomfort following each activation. The pain threshold may sometimes be exceeded so that a patient ceases to wear his appliance.

It is important not only to prevent these occurrences as far as possible but also to remedy the situation quickly. For this reason it is necessary to emphasize, preferably in written instructions, the importance of returning to the surgery for an emergency appointment. Appliances which are left out for any length of time may cease to fit and so require expensive and time consuming reconstruction. When circumstances prevent an early return for adjustment, the appliance should be worn for part of each day if possible.

Pain from the Teeth

From time to time a patient undergoing orthodontic treatment may complain of toothache. This pain need not necessarily be related to the wearing of an appliance.

Dental pain which proves to be of pulpal origin is likely to be merely coincidental to appliance wear. It is most unlikely that a removable appliance would apply sufficient pressure to devitalize a tooth, and should such a high force be applied then the appliance would be left out by the patient. Usually a history of trauma or the presence of a large restoration will point to the correct diagnosis. An X-ray may reveal arrested root development, or undetected caries. The remedy is to passify any springs acting on the affected tooth while root treatment is completed.

Occasionally an unsuspected cavity will become visible as orthodontic treatment proceeds and previously imbricated teeth begin to separate. Advantage may be taken of this and conservation carried out with excellent access. Subsequent orthodontic treatment will close the spaces and again restrict access.

The wearing of an orthodontic appliance may occasion dental pain which is of periodontal origin. Teeth may be sensitive to pressure from springs which have been over-activated or from clasps which are too tight. This occurs most commonly when an appliance has been recently fitted. The remedy is to reduce the pressure by appropriate adjustment.

Soft Tissue Pain

Trauma to soft tissues is a common source of difficulty soon after an appliance has been activated and distortion of a spring by the patient may cause similar difficulties. Any component of the appliance may be a source of trauma.

Trauma from the clasps. When arrowheads engage too deeply into the undercuts they may push into the subgingival area and cause pain. Diagnosis is usually straightforward as the pressure causes local tissue blanching. Adjustment of the clasps as described in Chapter 8 will relieve the discomfort.

Occasionally, despite the patient's complaint, tissue blanching is not seen and the clasp appears to be correctly adjusted. If this is the case then it is important to look at

156

the clasp with the teeth in occlusion. Sometimes an opposing tooth will occlude on a clasp arm as it passes over the contact point and so drive the arrowhead into the gingival margin. The remedy in this case is to re-contour the wire across the contact point and this is not always an easy procedure.

When headgear is used tubes soldered onto clasps may be the source of discomfort. They may stand proud buccally or the tube ends may not have been chamfered and smoothed. Face bows occasionally project too far beyond the distal of the tubes. Attention to the correct placement and adjustment of tubes and face bows should prevent these occurrences.

Trauma from springs. Springs acting from the buccal side undoubtedly cause more trouble than palatal ones. The problems arise as a result of faulty design and construction, or incorrect adjustment. Even a satisfactory spring can subsequently be distorted by a patient who uses the spring to remove the appliance.

Palatal springs are less likely to be distorted especially if they are protected by guardwires. Where successive teeth are being moved along the arch it is possible for a palatal spring which has completed its task to be trapped as the next tooth moves into contact. This occurs particularly when premolars are being moved distally and can be avoided by removing the first spring just before contact occurs.

It is important that the patient has the opportunity to wear the appliance at all times. Wires which cause trauma will make co-operation difficult and should, therefore, be adjusted at the earliest opportunity. If circumstances do not allow this then the dental surgery assistant may be able to help by giving or posting to the patient a quantity of soft carding wax. A small piece of this wax may be applied over an offending spring to make the appliance comfortable enough to wear for at least part of the time until an appointment can be arranged. This procedure will preserve the fit of the appliance and prevent unwanted tooth movement.

Trauma from the base plate. The base plate is not a common source of trouble and difficulty is generally only encountered during overjet reduction. If the acrylic is not adequately trimmed then mucosa palatal to the upper incisors may be compressed between the moving teeth and the base plate.

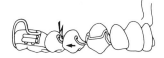

An occasional but irritating difficulty. The palatal spring has become trapped by movement of an adjacent tooth.

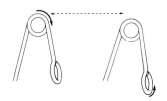

A buccal spring which extends too far into the sulcus may be adjusted by 'rolling' the coil down the posterior arm. The anterior arm is thus lengthened but may be shortened and readapted.

ANCILLARY PROBLEMS

Oral Hygiene

Removable appliances are much less likely than fixed appliances to damage the teeth and supporting structures. Nevertheless, attention to oral hygiene is still an important part of the management of orthodontic patients. Adequate patient education is essential at the commencement of treatment and in many cases a visit to the hygienist is wise. Deterioration of oral hygiene during treatment may necessitate re-instruction. Persistently poor oral hygiene may indicate that treatment should be abandoned.

Persistent Gagging

Fortunately this is a rare condition. Occasionally a patient seems unable to tolerate the presence of an appliance in the mouth. The first appliance should be designed to be as simple as possible and if it has a reduced area of palatal cover the patient may be able to get used to wearing it. Even if the appliance cannot be worn in the surgery it is helpful to let the patient take it home in order to attempt gradually increased periods of wear. A well-fitting appliance with the base plate firmly applied to the vault of the palate is essential.

Most of these problems are apparently psychogenic. Certainly a patient who masters the first appliance is likely to cope rapidly with any subsequent ones.

Specific Difficulties

Certain tooth movements give rise to a disproportionate number of difficulties:

Overbite Reduction

Many operators experience difficulty in achieving satisfactory overbite reduction. The commonest cause is inadequate appliance wear. Many patients will cope well with all aspects of appliance wear but will persistently remove the appliance to eat. In this way tooth movements with springs may progress well, but overbite reduction will be slow. Faulty adjustment of the bite plane is frequently responsible but careful adjustment as described in Chapter 2 will allow the patient to cope with the appliance full time.

Overbite reduction in Class II, division 2 malocclusions can be difficult so that it is advisable to start treatment in the actively growing patient wherever bite opening is required. Adult patients are similarly slow to respond to bite plane therapy and some cases may be totally unsuccessful in this respect. It is wise to be cautious in planning adult treatment which is based on overbite reduction.

Crossbite Correction

A unilateral posterior crossbite should respond readily to suitable removable appliance therapy provided there is a lateral mandibular displacement. Any difficulty experienced with this tooth movement can usually be attributed to faulty appliance design. Midline expansion puts great stress on appliance retention so that at least four clasps should be incorporated. During the course of treatment these clasps will require adjustment if retention is to be maintained. Occlusal interference from the lower arch may be a factor in slow progress either by limiting movement in the upper arch or by bringing about unwanted lower arch expansion. The addition of posterior bite planes will eliminate this problem.

Overjet Reduction

Unsatisfactory progress during overjet reduction is usually related to poor control of overbite. During the first stage of treatment the overbite reduction may be inadequate to permit subsequent overjet reduction before the upper and lower incisors make contact. Alternatively careless trimming of the bite plane during overjet reduction may allow the overbite to relapse partially or completely before the upper incisors achieve their correct position in relation to the lower incisors and lips. Careful attention to the procedures described in Chapter 2 should avoid these difficulties.

The Correction of Incisor Crossbite

This procedure is often used as an example of the simplest type of tooth movement. Frequently this is so, but there may be unexpected pitfalls, particularly in the treatment of upper lateral incisors. The overbite may be inadequate at the start or may rapidly become so as proclination occurs. Occasionally upper lateral incisors may occlude lingual to the cusps of lower canines which are themselves crowded mesially and labially. This can be difficult to resolve. The addition of posterior bite planes to the appliance may allow

159

the lower canines to align following lower premolar extractions. Otherwise a lower fixed appliance may be required.

RELAPSE

Virtually any corrected tooth must be maintained in the new position if stability is to be assured. Such stability can only be achieved if the new tooth position is likely to be maintained by the forces of occlusion and the soft tissue environment. It is unlikely that a Class II, division 2 malocclusion treated by the proclination of upper central incisors will ever be stable. Similarly, the proclination of lower incisors is frequently followed by relapse. If the general principle of moving teeth into new and potentially stable positions is observed most tooth movements will become stable quite quickly. Certain tooth movements, however, are associated with a strong tendency to relapse. It is important to recognize these and plan appropriate retention. Much local relapse can be traced to the influence of the periodontal tissues, in particular the free gingival and transeptal fibres.

Midline Spaces

It is common for a patient to request the reduction of an upper midline diastema in an occlusion which is otherwise acceptable. The necessary tooth movement is, of itself, usually straightforward, but as the central incisors are approximated spaces must appear further round the arch. Although it may be aesthetically acceptable to thus redistribute the space the probability of relapse is high. Two factors probably contribute to this. Firstly there may be an accumulation of soft tissue in the mid-line which, being under compression, tends to displace the central incisors distally. Secondly, the transeptal fibres connecting neighbouring teeth are placed under tension. Long retention is necessary as it is likely to take in excess of one year for the periodontal tissues to adapt. Gingival surgery such as gingivoplasty, fraenectomy or pericision will reduce this tendency to relapse.

Rotation

Rotation is probably the tooth movement with the highest rate of relapse. It seems probable that the free gingival fibres are responsible. Careful long-term retention, or pericision will reduce the extent of this relapse.

Single Outstanding Teeth

A single proclined tooth which has been retracted shows a high tendency to relapse. This may be related to occlusal interference from lower incisors which are preventing perfect alignment of the upper teeth and thus prejudicing their stability. It is likely that the displacement of gingival tissue may also play a part in this. Careful long term retention is essential.

Overjet

Partial reduction of overjet is a common cause of subsequent relapse. This may be due to deliberate partial reduction because the parent becomes concerned by increasing retroclination of the upper incisors. This is due to poor case selection. The underlying skeletal pattern is too severe for simple treatment.

Space assessment may be at fault. The operator may have failed to realize how much space full overjet reduction would require.

Faulty anchorage control is a very common cause of partial overjet reduction. Many dentists do not pay sufficient attention to this most important aspect of appliance management.

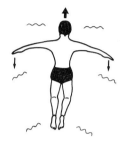

Distal movement of any teeth will exert a forward force on the anchor teeth. Where space is at a premium anchorage control must be given careful attention.

Class II, division 2 Malocclusions

Proclined lateral incisors in this malocclusion are, like any single outstanding tooth, very liable to relapse after correction. In addition to the factors discussed above, this may be associated with the mesio-labial rotation, and the mesial inclination which these teeth often demonstrate. These factors make perfect alignment difficult. While a satisfactory aesthetic result may be achieved the minimal residual irregularity may permit the displacing factors of occlusion and soft tissue forces to bring about a relapse.

Whenever long term retention is deemed necessary, it is worthwhile considering the provision of a specially constructed retainer. This has the advantage of simplicity, accurate fit and rigidity. It can be planned specifically to resist the anticipated pattern of relapse. In this respect it will be superior to a working appliance which has been passified.

Appendix

It is useful to reinforce verbal information with simple printed instructions. The following two examples may serve as models.

HEADGEAR

You have now been given a special kind of orthodontic appliance commonly known as 'headgear'. Although this looks very strange, particularly when you first see it, it offers great advantages in improving and speeding up your treatment. It is intended to be worn only when at home, rather than throughout the day like most other appliances, and you should very quickly get used to the unusual appearance. In order to reposition the front teeth, it is sometimes necessary to move back the teeth at the side of the mouth, and to do this we have to apply a 'pull' on these teeth from the back of the head.

Unless otherwise instructed, you are expected to fit the headgear early in the evening after your evening meal, wear it throughout the evening and during the night while you are in bed, and remove it in the morning before breakfast. It would speed up treatment if you could wear your headgear more than this, which means at weekends and holidays it could be worn during the normal day.

If the teeth are being moved satisfactorily with this appliance, they will feel slightly tender in the morning on first waking, but this tenderness should not last more than a few minutes after removing the appliance. Similarly, the teeth may feel very slightly loose when compared with the other teeth and this, like the tenderness, is a sign of teeth that are moving properly. You are expected to wear the headgear long enough and with enough pressure from the elastics to reach this stage.

162

Finally we would like you to keep a careful record of the hours you wear this part of your orthodontic appliance so that we may discuss this at each visit. You are personally responsible for the wearing of this headgear, and unless you co-operate fully with this your treatment will be unnecessarily prolonged.

REMOVABLE ORTHODONTIC APPLIANCES

A removable orthodontic appliance is normally intended to be worn full-time, and only removed from the mouth to be cleaned after taking food.

When first fitted the appliance will naturally feel strange and is likely to interfere with speaking and eating. This should pass off within a day or so, and should scarcely be noticeable thereafter.

This appliance must be treated carefully. It rarely breaks whilst in the mouth, but if carelessly handled outside the mouth is fairly easily damaged. Removal and replacement for cleaning purposes is straightforward but may be difficult at first. During the initial period it may be helpful to use a mirror, resting the elbows on a solid object such as a washbasin or table.

Cleaning the appliance should present no problem as most foods will readily wash off using water and a toothbrush. Sticky foods, toffee and chewing gum are more difficult and should be completely avoided.

The teeth must be kept thoroughly clean while treatment continues. At school, where cleaning may be difficult, the mouth and appliance should be rinsed with water.

In the event of the appliance becoming impossible to wear for any reason, such as breakage or pain, it should be left out. Do not wait until the next appointment, but telephone for an earlier appointment at once. If an appliance is left out for more than a few days, it may be impossible to adjust it to refit the mouth.

If it is necessary to remove an appliance for a time, for instance if it causes discomfort, or because you have been instructed not to wear it full-time, then put it in a plastic box or tin and not simply in the pocket.

The speedy success of treatment depends on the patient, so once again here are the important features:

1. Wear it at all times unless instructed otherwise.

2. In the case of discomfort, tell us, we will put it right.

3. Keep the teeth and appliance clean.

4. Do not lose the appliance, you may have to pay for a replacement.

5. Visit your dentist regularly for inspections and any necessary dental treatment while under the care of the Orthodontic Clinic.

Index